Current Research in Oncology

1972

ACADEMIC PRESS RAPID MANUSCRIPT REPRODUCTION

Based on a series of lectures held at the
National Institutes of Health
Bethesda, Maryland
during January 1972

Current Research in Oncology

1972

Edited by

C. B. ANFINSEN
MICHAEL POTTER
ALAN N. SCHECHTER

National Institutes of Health
Bethesda, Maryland

ACADEMIC PRESS 1973 New York and London

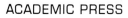

ACADEMIC PRESS, INC.
111 Fifth Avenue, New York, New York 10003

United Kingdom Edition published by
ACADEMIC PRESS, INC. (LONDON) LTD.
24/28 Oval Road, London NW1

Library of Congress Cataloging in Publication Data
Main entry under title.

Current research in oncology, 1972.

"Based on a series of lectures held at the National
Institutes of Health, Bethesda, Maryland during January
1972."
1. Oncology--Addresses, essays, lectures.
I. Anfinsen, C. B., ed.   II. Potter, Michael, ed.
III. Schechter, Alan N., ed.   [DNLM: 1. Neoplasms.
2. Research. QZ 206 O976 1973]
RC254.C87   616.9'92   72-88373
ISBN 0-12-058752-1

CONTENTS

CONTRIBUTORS

Edward A. Boyse
> Sloan-Kettering Institute for Cancer Research, New York, New York 10021

J. E. Cleaver
> Laboratory of Radiobiology, University of California, San Francisco, California 94122

Walter Eckhart
> The Salk Institute for Biological Studies, San Diego, California 92112

Emmanuel Farber
> Departments of Pathology and Biochemistry, Temple University School of Medicine, Philadelphia, Pennsylvania 19140

Robert W. Miller
> Epidemiology Branch, National Cancer Institute, National Institutes of Health, Bethesda, Maryland 20014

O. H. Pearson
> Department of Medicine, Case Western Reserve University, School of Medicine, Cleveland, Ohio 44106

Herbert J. Rapp
> Biology Branch, National Cancer Institute, National Institutes of Health, Bethesda, Maryland 20014

Philip S. Schein
> Medicine Branch, National Cancer Institute, National Institutes of Health, Bethesda, Maryland 20014

PREFACE

This collection represents the sixth set of lectures designed to review subjects of general and active interest in biomedical research for the large, diverse audience of scientists at the National Institutes of Health. The response at this institution to all of these lectures has been very gratifying, and the undiminishing interest of the heterogeneous audience seemed the best evidence for their general value as an educational device. It was, therefore, decided to publish these lectures for the use of physicians and research scientists, both here and elsewhere. A previous series of lectures given at the National Institutes of Health in September of 1971 has appeared in a volume entitled "Current Topics in Biochemistry."

The present volume is based on the series of lectures on various aspects of oncology, given in January of 1972. They were held at a time when a greatly increased national effort in cancer research was being widely discussed. The aim of these lectures was to provide an overview of a broad field of investigation for a diverse scientific audience. Speakers, selected for their eminence in particular areas of research in oncology, were asked to present general surveys and to integrate such backgrounds with their own work. The lectures dealt with a variety of specialties: etiology, epidemiology, pathogenesis, and therapy.

Quite independent of the increased public interest in the problems of oncology, the field itself appears to be undergoing major scientific transitions. First, the quest for a single unifying etiology, pathogenetic mechanism, and therapy seems to be all but replaced by the acceptance of the idea of a multiplicity of etiologic agents (viral, chemical, physical), pathogenetic mechanisms, and therapies. Underlying this change in attitude is the fact that tumors are as different from each other as are the different cell types within the organism. Since each tissue appears to have its own controls for regulating regeneration, cellular proliferation and orientation, the abnormalities of growth must be defined in terms of the parent tissue. Though a single therapy has been long sought it also appears that approaches to therapy are benefited by taking advantage of the special differentiation characteristics of each tumor cell.

A second transition in oncology is the ever-increasing interdependence of tumor research on the more basically oriented biological disciplines and, concomitantly, the greater frequency with which scientists trained in these areas are drawn to intriguing problems in oncology. In the past, many were reluctant to enter the area of oncology because of a pervading mystique surrounding the abnormal process. As basic information on the normal physiology of cells increases, the nature of the neoplastic disorder becomes a more easily approachable problem.

The physiology and molecular biology of the outer cell surface is one example of an area of interdependence. A major derangement in neoplastic cells is their ability to grow in environments other than those in which their normal counterparts are found. It is generally thought that the cell orientation is regulated by specific receptors on the cell surface. Abnormalities in the integrity of cell membrane and its receptors could lead to the phenomenon of neoplasia. One cannot help but be impressed with the extraordinary recent development of knowledge concerning the cell surface. The impact of this information on both the basic disciplines, as well as oncology itself, has been impressive and one realizes, in 1972, how great will be the acceleration of the attack on the cancer problem when further basic physiological information accumulates.

Once again, we are very grateful to Mrs. Anne Ettinger and Mrs. Dorothy Stewart of the Laboratory of Chemical Biology, NIAMDD, for their skillful and essential help in the preparation of this book. We also wish to thank the staff of Academic Press for its cooperation in the production of this volume.

C. B. Anfinsen
M. Potter
A. N. Schechter

ETIOLOGY OF CANCER: EPIDEMIOLOGICAL STUDIES

Robert W. Miller

Epidemiology Branch
National Cancer Institute
National Institutes of Health
Bethesda, Maryland 20014

In 1952 an intern at Hiroshima University hospital asked a patient a seemingly naive question, and made an important discovery. The patient was 30 years old and had lung cancer. The intern asked him why, when he was so young, did he develop this neoplasm. The patient said that it was probably because he had worked for 16 months during the war at the mustard-gas factory 50 miles from Hiroshima. The intern and his professor thought this possibility deserved further study. They visited the factory and, although it had closed 8 years before, the smell of the gases manufactured there could easily be detected. They learned that protective clothing was often not worn, and a large proportion of the workers had severe respiratory symptoms during their employment and afterwards. They traced other workers until they found that among 500 men who manufactured mustard gas, 49 had died of respiratory cancer (33 histologically confirmed)(21).

This epidemiologic study began by looking backward into the history of a single patient. In this way an important contribution was made to our understanding of chemical carcinogenesis in man. The experience illustrates that epidemiologic research, in contrast to experimental studies, is usually observational rather than experimental. Epidemiologists must take things as they are rather than as they

might want them to be. They must wait for natural
circumstances to create opportunities, and then make
the most of them.

The Simplest Approach: Descriptive Studies

There are two main phases of epidemiology: descriptive and analytical. The descriptive approach--
a source of hypotheses--can provide new clues to the
origins of disease. It seeks peculiarities in the
distribution of illness according to such variables
as age, sex, race and geography.

Childhood peaks in occurrence. In this regard,
childhood cancer has revealed some features of interest when distributed by single year of age. If the
data are grouped by 5-year age-intervals, as for
adults, dynamic changes in rates that occur in childhood would be overlooked. Neuroblastoma, for example,
exhibits a peak frequency of diagnosis within the
first year of life. Other cancers that exhibit early
peaks in occurrence are Wilms' tumor, retinoblastoma,
primary carcinoma of the liver, ependymoma, and leukemia (13). The occurrence of peaks, so soon after
birth, indicates that a large proportion, if not all
of these tumors have their origins either prezygotically (genetically) or during intrauterine life as
a consequence of environmental influences.

Ethnic differences. Leukemia shows another
feature of particular interest. When study is made of
the age distribution by ethnic group, the sharp peak
in mortality at 4 years of age observed among white
children, 1950-59, is not found among non-white children in the United States. The peak among whites is
due to variation in the frequency of acute lymphocytic leukemia. One must conclude that non-white children are either not exposed or not susceptible to an
agent that induces acute lymphocytic leukemia (but
not the myelogenous form of the disease)(13).

Another striking ethnic difference in cancer
occurrence is the near-absence of Ewing's sarcoma
among U.S. blacks, who show no such difference from

whites with respect to osteogenic sarcoma (7). This finding is of clinical value in the differential diagnosis of bone lesions affecting blacks, and is of research value in considering the origins of Ewing's tumor as distinguished from osteosarcoma.

Sex, size and bone sarcoma. A useful clue to the origin of bone sarcoma has come from veterinary medicine. The relative risk of bone sarcoma among giant breeds of dogs, such as the St. Bernard and the Great Dane, is about 200 times that for small- or medium-size breeds (20). This observation is consistent with the similarity in man between the patterns of growth (stature) and mortality rates for bone cancer (13). The average height by single year of age for boys and girls rises progressively and is virtually identical until 13 years of age, when boys grow taller than girls. Mortality rates for bone cancer are virtually identical for both sexes until precisely the same age, 13 years, when the rates for boys first exceed those for girls. These observations in both dogs and children suggest that the occurrence of bone sarcoma is closely related to the rate of bone growth.

Hodgkin's disease. Unlike the childhood cancers described above, the occurrence of bone sarcoma exhibits a gradual rise rather than an early peak. The same is true for mortality from Hodgkin's disease, but its age distribution shows an unusual feature. At 11 years, the rates which were climbing slowly make a discernible upward turn and rise to the first peak characteristic of this disease at 25-29 years of age (15). Since survival time is on the average 2.7 years, the upturn in diagnosis must have been at 8 years of age. One must then think what change in the environment or the host might be responsible. No suspicion falls heavily on any environmental agent at this time. With regard to susceptibility of the host, however, it is of interest that perhaps the largest physiological change just before 8 years of age is a tremendous involution of the lymphatic tissues (e.g., tonsils and adenoids). This involution, if faulty, might predispose to Hodgkin's disease, an ailment in which a substantial number of immunological abnormalities has been found.

Etiologic Value of Case-Histories

Another epidemiologic approach, retrospective or looking-backward studies, has been much maligned by the uninitiated. Yet some of the best leads in cancer etiology have come from this approach. There can be no more dramatic example than the cluster of adenocarcinoma of the vagina among young women at one hospital in Boston (17). This neoplasm is extremely rare so early in life, and the cluster could not be attributed to chance. Looking back into the history of 8 patients revealed that in 7 the mothers had been given stilbestrol during pregnancy because of threatened abortion. The relationship to the drug was quickly confirmed by a search of the New York State Tumor Registry, which revealed 5 more cases. Studies are now in progress to determine if stilbestrol during pregnancy induces other cancers or disorders of the offspring, and to determine if other drugs may do the same.

This is the first instance of transplacental carcinogenesis in man. The latent period was 14-22 years. Had a more common neoplasm, such as lymphoma or neuroblastoma been involved, the excess of cases probably would not have been noticed.

Chemical carcinogenesis. As indicated by the mustard-gas story, occupational cancers are recognized by retrospective study or by the occurrence of a cluster of cases within a factory or industry. Table 1 summarizes the cancers having the best evidence for induction by occupational exposures, as compared with those having the best evidence for drug-induction. It will be noted that much more has been learned about chemical carcinogenesis in man from occupational studies than from investigations into drug usage. The organs affected are also different for the two categories of exposure. Occupational cancers affect the respiratory tract, skin or urinary

TABLE 1

Cancers Due to Occupational Exposures (2), as Compared with Drug-Induction (6).

Occupational Chemical Carcinogenesis		Drug-Induced Cancer	
Asbestos	Lung Mesothelium	Prenatal synthetic estrogens	Adenocarcinoma, vagina
Nickel	Lung Paranasal sinuses	Phenacetin-containing drugs	Renal pelvis
Chromates	Lung	Chloramphenicol	Leukemia (?)
Arsenic	Lung (?) Skin	Melphalan Cyclophosphamide	Acute myelomonocytic leukemia (?)
Mustard gas	Respiratory tract	Diphenylhydantoin	Lymphoma (?)
Coke-ovens	Lung	Immunosuppressive drugs	Skin, lymphoma, other (?)
Woodwork	Nasopharynx	Radioactive drugs	Organs where concentrated
Chimney sweeps Tar workers Cotton spinners	Skin Scrotum	Arsenic	Skin of palms
α or β Naphthylamine	Urinary bladder	Chlornaphazine	Urinary bladder
Benzidene	Urinary bladder		
4-Aminobiphenyl	Urinary bladder		
Benzene	Leukemia		

5

system, and are due to breathing, touching or concentrating carcinogens. In response to drugs, cancers occur not only in the same organs as are affected by occupational exposures, but also in the lymphoreticular system. Drugs are, of course, ingested or applied topically. Cancers related to occupation or drugs tend to follow heavy prolonged exposures.

Need for record-linkage. Occupational studies have been valuable but under present circumstances they are usually slow, tedious and expensive. Many steps are involved, with considerable invasion of privacy. To locate subjects in the study after an interval of years, the epidemiologist has to contact relatives, neighbors, credit bureaus, the police and others. Follow-up would be immensely simplified if records could be linked more effectively. In some countries there are data resources that make it possible to link employment records, for example, with subsequent health data from hospital charts, insurance records or death certificates. In other countries, such as the United States, the establishment of a National Death Index could reduce follow-up from 30 or more steps to 3 primary steps: 1) obtain employment rosters from a specific industry for some time in the past--perhaps 20 or 30 years ago; 2) match the employment rosters against the National Death Index to determine the place and occurrence of death in subsequent years (a unique number, such as the Social Security number for each person would aid in the matching); and 3) obtain death certificates from the usual sources. The National Institute for Environmental Health Sciences is playing an important role in encouraging the establishment of the Index.

Cohort Studies

Matching records for a cohort of persons in the past against more recent records falls into the category of prospective studies--looking-forward studies. Once a relationship between cancer and a prior event is known or strongly suspected, following a cohort

through time will reveal such details of cancer occurrence as dose effects, age effects, and latent period.
Prospective studies can yield precise estimates of
risk. One example concerns radiation-induced leukemia
(16). The relationship was known from case-series and
from studies of the frequency of the neoplasm among
radiologists as compared with other physicians. After
the atomic bombs exploded in Japan cohorts of survivors were studied to determine delayed effects of radiation exposure. Excesses were soon noted in the
frequencies of acute leukemia and chronic myelogenous
leukemia, but notably not chronic lymphocytic leukemia. Clearly, radiation did not induce all forms
of leukemia equally. Presumably different etiologic
factors are involved. A dose-response effect was
noted, and a peak in the excess of leukemia occurred
in 1951, 6 years after exposure. The acute leukemias
continue to occur excessively, but chronic myelogenous
leukemia does not.

Clues from Concurrent Disease

Retrospective--looking backward; prospective--
looking forward; logic suggests a third category,
laterospective studies--looking sideways for collat-
eral disease. Recognizing an excess of cancer in persons with specific preexistent diseases provides an
opportunity to examine the etiology of a neoplasm in
the light of what is known of the etiology of diseases with which it is associated.

The excess of leukemia in children with Down's
syndrome is now well known. Since Down's syndrome is
determined prezygotically, through meiotic nondisjunc-
tion, the excess of leukemia among these children must
to some extent be prezygotically determined. It has
since been noted that with one exception all groups
with high risk of leukemia have preexistent cytogenic
abnormalities (14). Thus, in Fanconi's aplastic
anemia and in Bloom's syndrome there is genetically
induced chromosomal fragility on culture, in poly-
cythemia vera there are various preexistent chromosomal aberrations, and, following exposure to radia-

7

tion or benzene, there are long-persisting chromosomal
abnormalities. All of these conditions, either inborn
or acquired, carry a high risk of leukemia.

Persons with high probability of developing leukemia do not carry a similar risk of lymphoma, a neoplasm which is associated instead with inborn, immunological, cell-mediated deficiencies (congenital thymic
alymphoplasia, Wiskott-Aldrich syndrome and ataxia-
telangiectasia)(3). Thus the constellation of diseases
associated with leukemia are different from those
associated with lymphoma.

In an entirely different orbit are Wilms' tumor,
adrenal cortical neoplasia and primary liver cancer,
which are associated with several congenital growth
excesses (13). Each of the 3 neoplasms occurs excessively with congenital hemihypertrophy; the neoplasms and hemihypertrophy are independently associated
with large pigmented or vascular nevi, among other
hamartomas, and with the visceral cytomegaly syndrome
to which Beckwith has called attention (1). The syndrome consists of omphalocele, macroglossia and cytomegaly of visceral organs including the 3 in which
neoplasia has been observed in association with hemihypertrophy. Thus 4 manifestations of abnormal growth
are associated with one another: malignant neoplasms,
benign neoplasms, cytomegaly, and hemihypertrophy.

It should be noted that the malformations associated with leukemia, lymphoma and Wilms' tumor are
quite different, with very little overlap among them.
Leukemia is associated with preexistent chromosomal
abnormalities, lymphoma with immunosuppression, and
Wilms' tumor with various manifestations of growth
abnormality. Neuroblastoma, by contrast, falls into
none of these constellations, since comparable studies
have revealed no excessive occurrence with congenital
anomalies. These observations can be useful in identifying circumstances of the host or of the environment
that carry high risk of these neoplasms. The information is of value not only in prevention, but also can
be used by laboratory scientists to further the understanding of the relationship between oncogenesis and
teratogenesis.

Family Studies

A few words should be said about family studies. Increasingly an excessive aggregation of cancer in families is being recognized. The cancer may be of a single site, as in a Boston family in which 7 and possibly 10 women had ovarian cancer (10). Cancers of certain dissimilar cell types may also occur excessively in families. Familial cancer syndromes include one characterized by soft-tissue sarcomas in children and breast cancer, often in the mother, but also among other female relatives (8,9). The recurrence of the pattern and the rarity of some of the cell types strongly suggest that such family aggregates are not due to chance, although formal statistical proof of the excess in families may be difficult to achieve.

When such families are identified, studies of various members using newly developed laboratory techniques may reveal healthy members with subclinical abnormalities that portend the occurrence of cancer. A dramatic example is a family studied at NIH in which 6 members had acute myelogenous leukemia (including 3 in one sibship) and 2 had reticuloendotheliosis. Infection of skin fibroblasts in culture with SV 40 revealed increased "malignant" transformation in the only surviving child with leukemia, in a healthy sib, and in the mother, but not in the father (19). The distribution of cancer in the family, as well as the fibroblast transformation tests, indicated that the predisposition to neoplasia was transmitted through the maternal line.

Prenatal Origins of Some Cancers

By going over the data already presented and adding a little more, one can see to what extent cancer is prenatally determined (17). Prenatal determinants in which the mode of transmission is known may involve a) germ cells--genetic as in retinoblastoma or von Recklinghausen's disease, or cytogenetic as in the association between leukemia and Down's syndrome; b) transplantation--metastases from mother to child or from one identical twin to the other while sharing the placental circulation; c) ionizing radiation, an external agent that passes through the mother's abdominal wall to reach the fetus; and d) transplacental chemical induction, as noted above with regard to stilbesterol and adenocarcinoma of the vagina.

Other evidence of prenatal determinants in man involve observations for which the mode of transmission is unknown (17). They include the occurrence of a) congenital cancers, some of which grow to lethal size in utero; b) peaks in mortality soon after birth; c) the excessive concurrence of certain cancers with congenital malformations; and d) an increase in childhood leukemia related to high maternal age or low birth order.

Is Leukemia Infectious?

An important use of the epidemiologic technique is to test hypotheses. One hypothesis continually under review concerns the viral etiology of leukemia. If there is an infectious transmission, it might be detectable among persons having the closest contact with the neoplasm. Leukemia has not been found, however, to occur excessively among marital partners of leukemic persons or in children born of women with leukemia during pregnancy (12).

Leukemia in mice can be experimentally transmitted to the young by viruses in breast milk. Is there a human counterpart to this laboratory observation? The answer is no. The histories of children with leukemia revealed that as compared with neighborhood control children, there was no significant difference in the frequency or duration of breast-feeding (12).

The hypothesis that leukemia virus may be widely prevalent in blood but of low pathogenicity was evaluated by determining if children with leukemia were more often than usual exchange-transfused in the newborn period, when immunological defenses were low.

No significant difference between cases and controls was found in the frequency of neonatal exchange-transfusion (12).

An important development in cancer research has been the invention of statistical techniques for determining dispassionately whether the frequency with which a rare event clusters in time and space exceeds normal expectation (11). There is no doubt that, after examining the distribution of cases on a scatter map, one can identify individual clusters of rare diseases by inspection, and can draw tight boundaries around them. The question is not "Do rare events cluster?" but "Do they cluster excessively?" To date, the application of these new statistical procedures in studies of leukemia has provided no solid evidence of an excess suggesting an infectious mode of spread (4,5). In contrast, the application of one of these techniques to data for African lymphoma in the West Nile District of Uganda has shown considerable evidence of clustering (18). For this reason among others, an infectious origin is far more likely for African lymphoma than for leukemia.

These observations do not exclude the possibility of a viral role in leukemogenesis. They do indicate that, if viruses are involved, their mode of transmission is too subtle to be detected by the methods available at present--methods that have successfully revealed excesses of cancer following exposures to radiation or chemicals.

Interaction with Other Research Approaches

Epidemiology can either generate or test hypotheses. In so doing, a close interaction with laboratory observations is desirable. Epidemiologists should be aware of recent laboratory developments, and experimentalists should take into account epidemiologic findings in formulating their concepts based on laboratory studies.

11

References

1. Beckwith, J.B. Macroglossia, omphalocele, adrenal cytomegaly, gigantism, and hyperplastic viscero-megaly. Birth Defects: Original Article Series 5, 188 (1969).

2. Doll, R. Prevention of Cancer. Pointers from Epidemiology. London, England, Whitefriars Press Ltd., 1967.

3. Gatti, R.A. and Good, R.A. Occurrence of malig-nancy in immunodeficiency diseases. A literature review. Cancer 28, 89 (1971).

4. Glass, A.G., Mantel, N., Gunz, F.W. and Spears, G.F.S. Time-space clustering of childhood leu-kemia in New Zealand. J. Nat. Cancer Inst. 47, 329 (1971).

5. Fraumeni, J.F., Jr. and Miller, R.W. Epidem-iology of human leukemia: recent observations. J. Nat. Cancer Inst. 38, 593 (1967).

6. Fraumeni, J.F., Jr. and Miller, R.W. Drug-induced cancer. J. Nat. Cancer Inst. 48, 1267 (1972).

7. Jensen, R.D. and Drake, R.M. Rarity of Ewing's tumor in Negroes. Lancet 1, 777 (1970).

8. Li, F.P. and Fraumeni, J.F., Jr. Rhabdomyosar-coma in children: epidemiologic study and iden-tification of a familial cancer syndrome. J. Nat. Cancer Inst. 43, 1365 (1969).

9. Li, F.P. and Fraumeni, J.F., Jr. Soft-tissue sarcomas, breast cancer, and other neoplasms. A familial syndrome? Ann. Intern. Med. 71, 747 (1969).

10. Li, F.P., Rapoport, A.H., Fraumeni, J.F., Jr. and Jensen, R.D. Familial ovarian carcinoma. JAMA 214, 1559 (1970).

11. Mantel, N. The detection of disease clustering and a generalized regression approach. Cancer Res. 27, 209 (1967).

12. Miller, R.W. The viral etiology of leukemia: an epidemiologic evaluation. In Zarafonetis, C.J.D. (Ed.), Proceedings of the International Conference on Leukemia-Lymphoma. Philadelphia, Pennsylvania, Lea and Febiger, 1968.

13. Miller, R.W. Relation between cancer and congenital defects: an epidemiologic evaluation. J. Nat. Cancer Inst. 40, 1079 (1968).

14. Miller, R.W. Persons at exceptionally high risk of leukemia. Cancer Res. 27 Part 1, 2420 (1967).

15. Miller, R.W. Mortality in childhood Hodgkin's disease. JAMA 198, 1216 (1966).

16. Miller, R.W. Delayed radiation effects in atomic-bomb survivors. Science 166, 569 (1969).

17. Miller, R.W. Transplacental chemical carcinogenesis in man. J. Nat. Cancer Inst. 47, 1169 (1971).

18. Pike, M.C., Williams, E.H. and Wright. B. Burkitt's tumour in the West Nile District of Uganda 1961-5. Brit. Med. J. 2, 395 (1967).

19. Snyder, A.L., Li, F.P., Henderson, E.S. and Todaro, G.J. Familial acute myelogenous leukaemia: identification of possible inherited leukaemogenic factors in a kindred. Lancet 1, 586 (1970).

20. Tjalma, R.A. Canine bone sarcoma: estimation of relative risk as a function of body size. J. Nat. Cancer Inst. 36, 1137 (1966).

21. Wada, S., Miyanishi, M., Nishimoto, Y., Kambe, S. and Miller, R.W. Mustard gas as a cause of respiratory neoplasia in man. Lancet 1, 1161 (1968).

XERODERMA PIGMENTOSUM, DNA REPAIR AND CARCINOGENESIS[*]

J. E. Cleaver

Laboratory of Radiobiology
University of California
San Francisco, California 94122

This lecture will deal with three aspects of DNA repair and carcinogenesis:

(1) The main part will describe the features of a biochemical pathway for repair of genetic material (DNA) which is defective in a human hereditary disease that exhibits a high degree of carcinogenesis.

(2) Second, I would like to comment on DNA damage and repair from some chemical carcinogens.

(3) Third, and most briefly, I will comment on the insights into carcinogenesis that may be provided by this repair-deficient human disease.

Xeroderma Pigmentosum--Symptoms of the Disease-- Xeroderma pigmentosum (XP)(Fig. 1) is a rare human hereditary disease in which the skin is extremely sensitive to radiation of the short wavelength end of the sun's spectrum (below 3100 Å, approximately)(12). Sunlight produces skin cancers of both ectodermal and mesodermal origin (basal cell carcinomas, squamous cell carcinomas, melanomas, angiosarcomas, fibrosarcomas, and keratoacanthomas). The cancers develop on the sun-exposed areas during the first years of life and continually recur. When skin from an unexposed area is transplanted to the face, the typical progression on the transplanted skin consists of increased pigmentation, keratoses, and then malignancy.

---

[*] Work performed under the auspices of the U.S. Atomic Energy Commission.

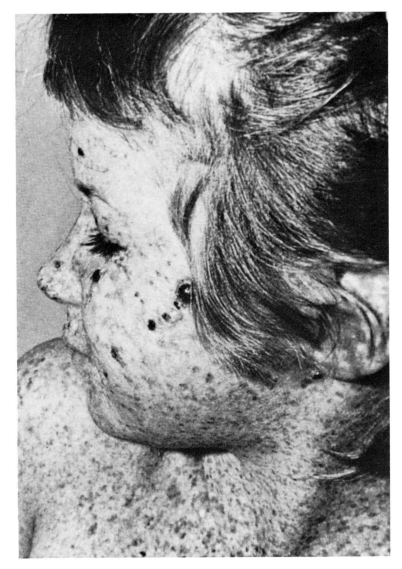

Fig. 1. Xeroderma pigmentosum patient.

Death often occurs early in life from metastases, unless careful palliative and preventative treatment is given. Hebra and Kaposi first identified the disease in 1874; they accurately described the malignancies

and suggested that the disease might be hereditary in
view of its appearance in early childhood. In a min-
ority of cases there are additional severe neurologi-
cal complications including microcephaly with mental
deficiency, premature closing of the epiphyses and
cranial sutures, cerebellar ataxis, retarded development, and adrenal and pituitary decline; this form is
named after those who first described it as the de
Sanctis Cacchione syndrome (Table 1). The two forms
have never been described within the same family.

TABLE 1

XERODERMA PIGMENTOSUM VARIANTS

	SYMPTOMS	BIOCHEMISTRY
XP, COMMON FORM	SKIN MALIGNANCIES	REDUCED EXCISION REPAIR
XP, DESANCTIS CACCHIONE	SKIN MALIGNANCIES, CENTRAL NERVOUS SYSTEM	REDUCED EXCISION REPAIR
XP, VARIANT	SKIN MALIGNANCIES	DNA REPAIR NOT INVOLVED
PIGMENTED XERODERMOID	MILD ACTINIC SKIN SENSITIVITY	DNA REPAIR NOT INVOLVED

Two other conditions also deserve mention. An XP
variant has recently been described in two unrelated
families in which the symptoms are indistinguishable
from the common form of XP, but the biochemistry appears to be quite different. A disease with mild
actinic skin sensitivity appearing in middle to late
age has been described by Jung (1970) and named "pigmented xerodermoid" (11). I am at present unconvinced
that this is a disease distinct from chronic sun-
damaged skin in a normal person. Except where expli-
citly mentioned, all that is said about XP will apply
equally to the common and the de Sanctis Caccione
forms.

The disease is inherited as autosomal recessive
gene without any obvious chromosomal abnormalities.
In one case of XP, however, German (10) has identified
a very small proportion of cells in fibroblast cultures

(2 to 3%) which have a balanced translocation (between groups 1 and D, or within group C). The general significance of this as a possible characteristic of XP remains to be established with other cases. The chromosomal rearrangement is, however, considerably smaller than that seen in some other hereditary diseases associated with malignancy in which the biochemistry of DNA repair is apparently normal (e.g., Blooms syndrome, Fanconi's anemia, and Louis-Barr syndrome or ataxia telangiectasia). Cells from patients with XP also have normal sensitivity to transformation with SV40 virus (1) unlike cells from some other diseases in which there are high levels of malignancy (e.g., Fanconi's anemia, Down's syndrome, and "high-sarcoma" families). Cultured cells have normal lifetimes *in vitro* and show no features of premature aging, although in several cases they have proven somewhat difficult to grow.

The potential value to cancer research arising from studies of XP is that in this disease extremely high rates of carcinogenesis are produced by UV light, an agent which can be precisely quantitated and whose biological effects are probably among the best understood of many physical or chemical agents. My own contribution in recent years has been to initiate identification of a biochemical defect which may play a role in the development of malignancy in a human disease (3-7).

Major Classes of DNA Damage and Repair Mechanisms-- Most kinds of damage (Fig. 2) to DNA involve only one strand of the molecule, either a broken phosphodiester chain or an altered base (e.g., cyclobutane pyrimidine dimer). Even some of the chemically induced cross-links between strands rarely involve both bases of a hydrogen bonded base pair. The redundancy of information in the complementary strands of DNA is thus a guarantee against the irretrievable loss of genetic information induced by radiations or chemical agents.

Most repair systems consist of biochemical pathways by which an intact double-stranded region of DNA is reconstructed from a region containing a damaged

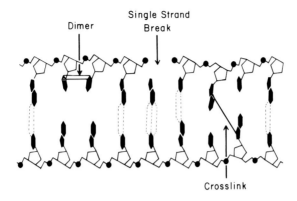

Fig. 2. Alterations in DNA caused by UV light (base damage: thymine dimers and cytosine hydrates) and ionizing radiation (chain breaks).

site on one of the strands. There are three major classes of repair systems in bacteria: photoreactivation, host cell reactivation (excision repair), and recombination (Table 2). Photoreactivation, a one-enzyme system that uses visible light as an activating agent, is specific for repair of the pyrimidine

TABLE 2

MAIN CLASSES OF DNA REPAIR SYSTEMS

	MECHANISM	SENSITIVE AGENTS
PHOTOREACTIVATION (PHR)	DIRECT REVERSAL	
EXCISION REPAIR (UVR, HCR)	REMOVAL AND RESYNTHESIS	UV, 4NQO, 8MOP, MIT-C
RECOMBINATION REPAIR (REC)	SYNTHESIS AROUND DAMAGE	UV, 4NQO, MIT-C, XRAYS, MMS, EMS, NTG

dimer but is completely absent from placental mammals and will concern us no further here. Host cell reactivation or excision repair involves the removal of damaged bases from DNA and synthesis of replacement regions. Recombinational repair involves repair of DNA strand breaks, semiconservative synthesis on

19

damaged templates, and strand exchange between paren-
tal and newly synthesized strands.

XP is a human mutation which is an analog of the
excision repair mutants designated UVRA, B, and C in
Escherichia coli, although a close parallel between
the human disease and the three distinct loci in *E.
coli* cannot yet be made. Jung (11) has claimed that
the pigmented xerodermoid condition is an analog of
the REC⁻ mutants, but the evidence thus far adduced
is not sufficient to prove the claim.

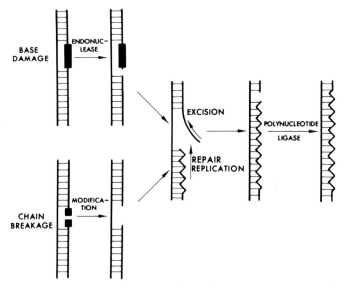

Fig. 3. Heuristic scheme for the steps in excision
repair of damaged bases and chain breaks by a common
pathway. The initial step for each kind of damage has
some unique features but the later stages can be common. (Reproduced from Cleaver [8].)

Tests for Excision Repair-- To demonstrate that
XP is a human analog of UVR⁻, the following experimental tests were made of the model for excision repair (Fig. 3):

(a) Are individual cells of XP genotype sensitive to UV light (6)?

(b) How well do XP fibroblasts support the growth of UV-damaged viruses (1,12)?

(c) Are thymine dimers formed and removed from DNA (5,13)?

(d) Are single strand gaps made and joined during excision?

(e) Are short regions of new bases inserted into DNA to replace excised dimers (2-6)?

(f) Are short regions of new bases inserted to repair single strand breaks (4,7)?

Sensitivity of Xeroderma Pigmentosum Cells-- The clinical symptom of XP patients is a high incidence of UV-induced skin cancers, but this could be due to a variety of systemic factors other than the inherent properties of individual cells. It is important to demonstrate that the XP genotype has some phenotypic expression in individual cells. The only method at our disposal is colony formation by single cells, but unfortunately primary fibroblasts have a low plating efficiency (a maximum of 10 to 20%). Use of this method presupposes that the cells that form colonies are a random sample of the population and are typical of the whole population in terms of their UV sensitivity. Granted these presuppositions, XP fibroblasts are much more sensitive than normal cells (Fig. 4). Certain of the XP cases recently identified have normal UV sensitivity (Fig. 4) which would exclude the involvement of any DNA repair system in these cases where normal levels of excision repair are also observed.

Host Cell Reactivation of UV-Damaged Viruses-- Some classes of UV-sensitive bacteria have a reduced ability to support the reproduction of UV-damaged phage, presumably because the same enzyme system repairs host DNA and infecting phage DNA. Experiments that illustrate this phenomenon in human cells have been done with herpes and SV40 virus (1)(Fig. 5) and XP fibroblasts appear to be analogs of bacteria that are defective in host cell reactivation.

Excision of Pyrimidine Dimers from Human Cells-- The number of dimers formed in the DNA of human cells

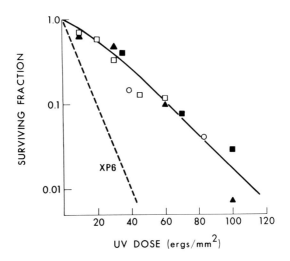

Fig. 4. Survival curve for human fibroblasts irradiated with UV light. Normal cells ▲, ■; XP variants with normal excision repair ◻, o; XP cells with low excision repair ----.

increases linearly with UV dose if the cells are fixed immediately after irradiation. When cells are allowed to grow for a time after irradiation before fixation and measurement, normal cells excise some of the dimers from their DNA, whereas XP cells apparently do not (Fig. 6). However, only about 50 to 75% of the dimers are excised from normal human cells, even at low UV doses. Bacteria are much more efficient in excision and some can excise nearly 100% of the dimers from their DNA. Finally, with respect to dimer studies, the assay is not sufficiently precise to distinguish between a low and a completely negligible excision level. Other studies make it likely that low levels of excision occur in XP cells.

Formation and Sealing of Single Strand Breaks during Dimer Excision-- The detection of small numbers of DNA strand breaks in animal cells is undoubtedly one of the most difficult technical problems in studies of DNA repair. If we did not know what sort of

22

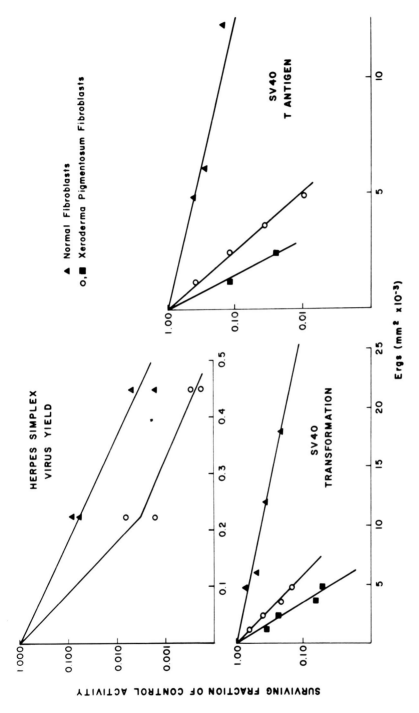

Fig. 5. Percentage of remaining virus activity of irradiated viruses grown on normal or XP cells. (Reproduced from Cleaver [8].)

23

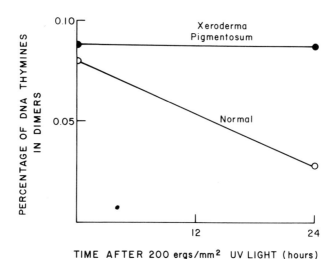

Fig. 6. Percentage of thymine-containing dimers in the acid insoluble fraction of normal and XP cells after irradiation with UV light.

answer we wanted, on the basis of dimer excision and repair replication experiments, I doubt that any of the studies of strand breaks during excision repair would be believed. The problem is that the number of breaks made during excision repair is small, and these breaks produce only a small change in the size of single strands that can be isolated from mammalian cells by alkaline sucrose gradient techniques (Fig. 7).

From the few studies made in human and bovine cells, we can fairly confidently say that excision repair appears to involve a relatively small number of strand breaks at any one time in relation to the number of dimers (about 10^4 per cell in contrast to about 10^6 dimers per cell at 100 ergs/mm^2 in bovine cells). One can therefore envisage repair proceeding by means of complex associations of enzymes which operate on a small proportion of the total number of lesions and move on sequentially from one lesion to another. The number of breaks is a measure of the number of lesions being repaired at any one time and

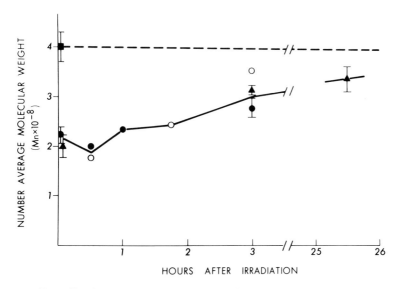

Fig. 7. Number-average molecular weight at various times after irradiation of bovine fibroblasts with UV light. Control ■, 100 ergs/mm^2 ●, 200 ergs/mm^2 ▲, 100 ergs/mm^2 grown in 10^{-3} M hydroxyurea after irradiation with 100 ergs/mm^2 o.

may indicate roughly the order of magnitude of enzyme complexes in a cell (i.e., 10^4).

Insertion of New Bases to Repair DNA-- Replacement of excised dimer-containing regions requires synthesis of very small amounts of DNA in short regions, "repair replication." This has to be detected in the presence of the relatively large amounts of semiconservative DNA replication that occur during the cell cycle.

Two methods can be used to distinguish repair replication from semiconservative replication. One method consists of using autoradiography to detect small amounts of radioactive thymidine (^{3}HTdR) incorporated into cells during repair replication when the cells are incapable of semiconservative replication. DNA repair detected in this way is called "unscheduled synthesis" (2,3) to distinguish it from normal

25

"scheduled" DNA synthesis that gives rise to heavily labeled cells. An elegant demonstration of such repair in normal skin, and its absence in XP skin, can be seen if ^{3}HTdR is injected intradermally soon after exposure of the skin to UV light (9)(Fig. 8).

From hybridization experiments in tissue culture it has been shown that cells from patients with the common form of XP and the de Sanctis Cacchione form can complement one another (6). In hybrid binucleate cells with one nucleus from each form of XP the level of unscheduled synthesis is indistinguishable from that in normal cells. This would suggest that the two forms of the disease represent different mutations that can complement one another either inter- or intragenically.

Repair Replication-- Another method for detecting repair replication takes advantage of the difference between the short pieces synthesized during repair and the long strands synthesized by semiconservative replication (3,5-7). Tritiated bromodeoxyuridine (^{3}HBrUdR, molecular weight 308) is used as a heavy analog of 3HTdR (molecular weight 242) and is incorporated into DNA in its place. The long chains formed by semiconservative replication are denser than normal and ^{3}H-labeled. The pieces synthesized by repair replication are such small patches in long molecules that the density of the molecules is unchanged, but they too will be ^{3}H-labeled. Thus, the presence of ^{3}H-labeled molecules of normal density is an indication that repair replication has occurred. DNA can be fractionated on the basis of its density by means of centrifugation through cesium chloride gradients (Fig. 9), which show that XP fibroblasts perform much less repair replication than normal cells. Most XP fibroblasts from donors in North America have residual repair capacity that is below 25% of normal (Table 3). Higher levels have been found in some Dutch cases (2) in which a correlation has also been established between the severity of the disease and the reduction of unscheduled synthesis. Most heterozygotes show normal repair levels although a few have been identified in

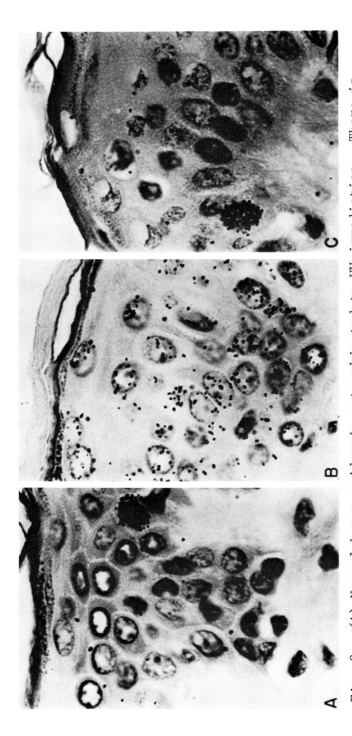

Fig. 8. (A) Normal human epidermis not subjected to UV irradiation. There is dense labeling of one basal cell in normal S-phase DNA synthesis. (B) Normal human epidermis irradiated with 13.6 x 10⁴ ergs/mm² UV light. There is sparse labeling of cells throughout the epidermis. (C) Epidermis of an XP patient irradiated with 13.5 x 10⁴ ergs/mm² UV light. There is one densely labeled basal cell but no sparse labeling. All skin was injected with 3HTdR (10 μCi/ml), from Epstein et al. [9]. Copyright 1970 by the American Association for the Advancement of Science.

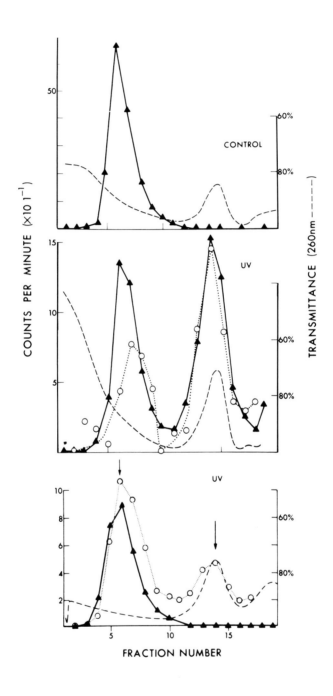

Fig. 9. Equilibrium density gradients from normal and XP cells irradiated with 200 ergs/mm^2 UV light and labeled for 4 hours with ^{3}HBrUdR. Arrows mark positions of normal density (1.698 gm/cc) and bromo-uracil substituted density (1.751 gm/cc). Dashed line indicates the total amount of DNA in the gradients (high values in the first few fractions are an artefact). *Top*, unirradiated normal cells. *Center*, normal (▲) and heterozygous XP (o) fibroblasts irradiated with 200 ergs/mm^2. Note the large peak of radioactivity at a density of 1.698 gm/cc which indicates repair replication. *Bottom*, two different fibroblast cultures, from unrelated homozygous XP patients, irradiated with 200 ergs/mm^2 UV light. Note the low repair replication peak at 1.698 gm/cc in one case (o) and the absence in the other (▲). (Reproduced from Cleaver [8].)

which reduced excision repair levels have been detected at moderate UV doses (greater than about 100 ergs/mm^2) (6).

Repair replication starts immediately after irradiation and most of the incorporation of new bases is complete within 3 to 5 hours in cultured cells, although some repair replication can still be detected 24 hours after irradiation (15 to 20% of initial rate)(Fig. 10).

Xeroderma Pigmentosum - Summary of Characteristics-- The accumulated evidence of the biochemical features of XP cells indicates that this human cell type is very similar to the bacterial strains that are designated UVR$^-$ and HCR$^-$. Both XP cells and these bacterial mutants are UV-sensitive and X-ray-resistant, have reduced abilities to excise UV photoproducts, and perform repair replication, but repair damage associated with DNA breaks at normal efficiency. Damage that is repaired to normal extents includes that from X-rays, methyl-methane sulfonate, and N-methyl-N'-nitro-nitrosoguanidine (7). Thus, it is probable that the biochemical defect in XP is in an enzyme associated with dimer excision such as an endonuclease.

TABLE 3

RELATIVE LEVELS OF EXCISION REPAIR (MEASURED DURING 4 HR AFTER 220 ERGS/MM^2 UV LIGHT, 254 NM).[*]

			Percent
Normal skin fibroblasts			100
Normal skin fibroblasts (SV40 transformed)			121
Fibroblasts (isolated by amniocentesis)			103
HeLa (cervical carcinoma)			94

Xeroderma pigmentosum

			Percent
Heterozygote	♀	XPH1	67,84,87
	♀	XPHK[§]	100
	♂	XPH11M	44,48
	♀	XPH11F	47,42
Homozygote		XPJ	6
		XP6	5.1,5.5
		XP7	5
		XP11	< 4
(SV40 transformed)		XP7	< 16
Homozygote		XP1[§][†]	9
		XP2[§][†]	25
		XPIW[§]	0
		XPKM[§][†]	0
		XPKF[§][†]	0

[*]Standard deviation is 20 percent of quoted value. (Upper limit cited when no distinct normal density ^{3}H peak was detectable in the isopycnic gradient.) (9)
[§]de Sanctis Cacchione syndrome. XP1,2 diagnosed by E. Klein, Roswell Park Institute. XPIW, KM, KF diagnosed by W. B. Reed, UCLA.
[†]Siblings.

The detection of at least two complementary defects in XP (the common form and the de Sanctis Cacchione syndrome) implies that either the enzyme in XP is a multiunit enzyme with subunits that have different functions, or that there are at least two enzymes involved. There are useful analogies to be made with bacteria in which at least three distinct genetic loci (UVRA,B,C) are associated with excision (Fig. 11).

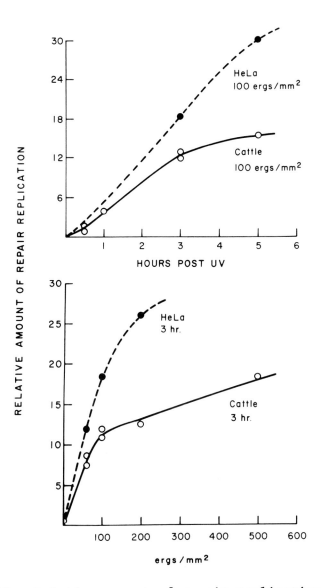

Fig. 10. Relative amount of repair replication determined from isopycnic gradients (cf. Fig. 9) as a function of UV dose and time after irradiation.

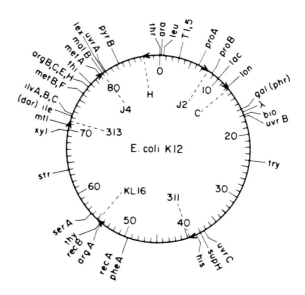

Fig. 11. Genetic map of *E. coli*; loci associated with excision repair are UVRA, UVRB, and UVRC.

Excision Repair and Inhibitors-- Since excision repair has many features that are biochemically different from semiconservative replication it is not surprising that the two kinds of replication respond in different ways to some inhibitors (Table 4). In particular, drugs whose main mode of action is on the metabolic pathways for synthesis of the precursors for replication inhibit semiconservative replication preferentially. This may be because of the small numbers of precursors required for excision repair in contrast to semiconservative replication.

The responses to drugs (Table 4) illustrate a distinct difference between excision repair in bacteria and animal cells. The drugs that bind to DNA (acriflavine, crystal violet, actinomycin D, and chloroquin) specifically inhibit excision repair in *E. coli* but inhibit semiconservative and repair replication equally in animal cells. Also, caffeine inhibits excision repair in *E. coli* possibly by affecting nucleases but inhibits semiconservative replication only in animal cells.

TABLE 4

INHIBITORS OF DNA SYNTHESIS

	INHIBITION OF DNA SYNTHESIS	
	Normal	Repair
METABOLIC INHIBITORS		
HYDROXYUREA 10^{-3}M	++	0
ARABINOSYL CYTOSINE 10^{-5}M	++	0
5 AMINOURACIL 5×10^{-3}M	++	0
FLUORODEOXYURIDINE 10^{-5}M	++	0
DNA BINDING AGENTS		
ACRIFLAVINE 5×10^{-5}M	++	++
CRYSTAL VIOLET 6×10^{-5}M	++	++
ACTINOMYCIN D 7×10^{-6}M	++	++
CHLOROQUIN 10^{-4}M	+	+
CAFFEINE 10^{-3}M	++	0
IODOACETATE 10^{-2}M	++	++
CYCLOHEXIMIDE 3×10^{-5}M	++	+

0 = no effect

+ = small effect ($<$50% inhibition)

++ = large effect ($>$50% inhibition)

These observations imply that excision repair and drug pharmacology are different in bacteria and animal cells. The use of microorganisms as a screening system for selecting drugs to use in combination with radiotherapy for cancer treatment could therefore be very misleading. Also, the use of inhibitors whose mode of action on repair is characterized in bacteria as a tool to elucidate details of repair in animal cells could be misleading.

Excision Repair, Patch Size and DNA Breakdown-- The size of the patch made by repair replication after UV damage is considerably larger than the dimer itself. Estimates based on the efficiency of photolysis of the BrU-containing patch, quantitation of unscheduled synthesis and repair replication, and fragmentation of repaired DNA all give values in the range from 50 to 500 bases. Of these estimates the lowest value is probably most accurate. Estimates of patch size indicate that there must be a small amount of excision of all bases around the dimer and repair replication should insert both pyrimidine and purine bases. Although repair replication can be detected with both thymidine and deoxycytidine, it has been difficult to detect with the purines, possibly because of the large variety of pathways into which purines can be diverted.

A major difference between bacteria and animal cells associated with excision is the very large amounts of DNA breakdown that occur in bacteria after UV irradiation. In contrast, very little DNA breakdown occurs in animal cells other than that arising from the destruction of lethally irradiated cells.

Comparisons of Excision Repair in Various Mammalian Species-- The excision repair system as seen in human and XP cells constitutes a dramatic example of the biological function and importance of a particular biochemical pathway. I must emphasize, however, that once one departs from this example and attempts to study excision repair in other mammalian cells, there are serious technical and theoretical questions that have to be faced in order to ascribe a similar role to the excision repair system. The correlation between the amount of excision repair and survival in normal and XP cells is unique. In general, the amount of repair replication increases not with the level of survival but with the level of killing. The more damage there is to DNA the more repair replication is detected. Consequently, much of what we call repair does not result in recovery from damage. Either it is ineffective repair or it involves only a proportion of the damaged sites or other competing degradative processes dominate at high levels of damage.

An even more serious question is raised by the failure of many investigators to detect excision of dimers in rodent cell lines, even when relatively high levels of repair replication occur (Table 5). We

TABLE 5

SENSITIVITY, DIMER EXCISION AND REPAIR
REPLICATION IN MAMMALIAN CELLS

	D_0 (ergs/mm^2)	EXCISION	REPAIR REPLICATION %*
PRIMARY HUMAN	30	YES	100
HeLa	108	YES	100
XP6	9	0	5
PRIMARY BOVINE	23	YES	60
PRIMARY MOUSE	—	—	100
MOUSE L CELLS	70–80	0	60
MOUSE ASCITES	700–800	0	—
CHINESE HAMSTER V79	43–50	0	100
CHINESE HAMSTER BFAF	60	0	10–20
PIG PS	210	0	—

*Expressed as percentage of human

might conclude from the evidence on dimer excision
that the rodents as a whole represent a situation similar to XP, but they do not exhibit high UV sensitivity.
Thus, either the failure to detect dimer excision in
rodents is due to a technicality or we must devise
new roles for repair replication and accept the possibility that the absence of excision repair may have no
functional significance in these animals. The latter,
if true, will make it particularly difficult to relate
the human results from XP with the extensive information on carcinogenesis based on rodents. But the most
probable resolution of this problem will come with
improved precision in detection of low levels of excision in rodent cells.

   DNA Repair and Carcinogens-- The incorporation
of new bases during repair provides an easy, rapid
technique for detecting the effect of agents that

cause damage to DNA, especially when using autoradio-
graphic procedures. Correlations can be made (15)
between the amount of unscheduled synthesis produced
by derivatives of the carcinogen 4-nitroquinoline-1-
oxide (4NQO) and the carcinogenic activities of these
derivatives (Fig. 12). 4 NQO acts by binding to guanine bases and producing a lesion in DNA that is han-
dled in a way closely resembling the handling of
pyrimidine dimers by excision repair. Thus, in this
family of derivatives, which presumably have qualita-
tively similar modes of action, the amount of unscheduled synthesis induced is indicative of the
amount of DNA damage caused by each derivative. The
damage is thus correlated with the carcinogenic activity. If we wish to relate this observation on chemical carcinogenesis with the radiation carcinogenesis
in XP, then we can say that in both situations the
carcinogenic potential is correlated with the amount
of damage to DNA. In the one case the amount of unscheduled synthesis indicates the amount of chemical
damage, of which only a portion may be repaired; in
the other the amount of unscheduled synthesis indicates the amount of initial damage that has been repaired.

Some comparisons can be useful in carefully considered situations. When, however, a variety of different, potentially carcinogenic agents are investigated, there is no guarantee that there will be any
correlation between unscheduled synthesis and carcinogenic activity. In fact there are good reasons why
one should not even expect such correlations.

The amount of unscheduled synthesis that one ob-
serves after treatment with any agent will depend not
only on the amount of damage to DNA but on its chemical nature and stability and on the manner in which
it is repaired. Some kinds of damage involve the insertion of large numbers of bases whereas other kinds
involve insertion of relatively few. Such contrasts
are readily seen in a comparison between the effects
of X-rays and UV light (Table 6). At the same levels
of killing and mutagenesis there are extremely large

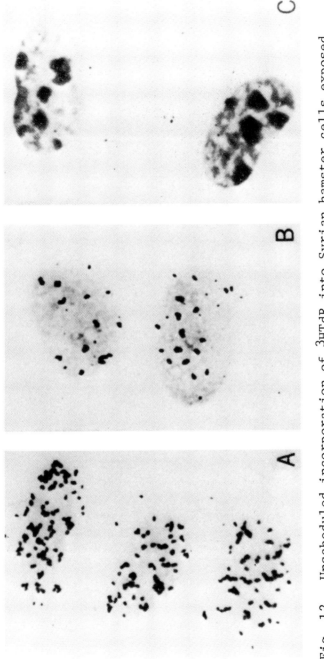

Fig. 12. Unscheduled incorporation of ^{3}HTdR into Syrian hamster cells exposed *in vitro* to the highly oncogenic 2-methyl-4NQO (A); the weakly oncogenic 8-methyl-4NQO (B); and the non-oncogenic 4-amino-quinoline (C); at a concentration of 10^{-5} M. (Reproduced from Stick, *et al.* [15].)

TABLE 6

LESIONS, MUTATIONS AND UNSCHEDULED

SYNTHESIS IN HUMAN CELLS

	Xrays	UV Light
D_o	100R	30 ergs/mm^2
Lesions	600 s.s. breaks 60 d.s. breaks 400 bases	2.5×10^5 dimers
Mutation rate	2×10^{-4}	3×10^{-4}
Unscheduled synthesis	180 (1 base/break)	6×10^6 (170 bases/excised dimer)

differences in the amounts of unscheduled synthesis; this difference is due to the small number of bases that are involved in repairing X-ray damage in contrast to UV damage. If mutation rate is any indication of the carcinogenic activity of an agent, then there is clearly no correlation between unscheduled synthesis and mutation (or carcinogenic) rates from UV light and X-rays. Thus, any comparison that is made between chemically disparate compounds in an attempt to predict carcinogenic activity on the basis of unscheduled synthesis is likely to be misleading.

Xeroderma Pigmentosum, DNA Repair and Carcinogenesis-- The most important aspect of XP and the one which first drew my attention to the disease has received little attention yet experimentally. This aspect is the outstanding clinical symptom of carcinogenesis. It has taken a considerable length of time to define the biochemical features of the disease adequately, and the implications of these features for carcinogenesis are something for speculation and future experiments. XP is, so far, a unique disease in its association between defective repair and carcinogenesis. Other malignant cells and diseases that have been studied with DNA repair in mind have shown normal DNA repair levels. Thus, if XP is unique in this regard, how does the disease fit into the general picture of carcinogenesis that may be beginning to take shape? Is it a special case which conveys no general message, or is it a pregnant example with much yet to produce?

The first question to be decided is whether the DNA repair defect is likely to have anything to do with the etiology of the disease. The existence of several XP variant cases with normal repair makes this question particularly pressing. We will, however, forget these cases for the time being until we can decide what to do with them. (Calling them a different disease would eliminate that little awkwardness in a manner that is not without precedent in medicine). If we conclude that the DNA repair defect has some relevance to the disease, this is at least a useful working hypothesis. Several lines of argument make this reasonable: the defective pathway is involved intimately with a major biological effect of the carcinogenic agent, there is a correlation between the severity of the disease and the extent of the biochemical defect, and two clinical forms of the disease have different complementary biochemical defects in repair.

Assuming, therefore, that defective DNA repair is somehow involved with UV carcinogenesis in XP, we can immediately exclude from consideration possibilities such as radiation damage increasing the permeability of receptor sites of the cell membrane to oncogenic viruses. Unrepaired lesions in the human cell DNA which thereby alter a cell's genetic information potentiate the chances of carcinogenesis in XP. To assess the possible implication of this we should first turn to *E. coli* again and consider the properties of UVR⁻ strains, the mutant strains analogous to XP. In response to UV damage these strains show an elevated mutation rate in many loci and also a reduction in the dose needed for induction of lysogenic phage. We might expect both phenomena to occur also in XP cells, which gives us two alternatives to consider in relation to carcinogenesis. In animal cells there are several reports which indicate that irradiation of the host cell causes an increase in the transformation rate by oncogenic viruses, although with UV light the increase is only relative to cell survival; there is a decrease in the absolute number of transformed cells.

There are, then, at least three alternatives, not necessarily mutually exclusive, by which we can consider the mechanism of carcinogenesis in XP: increased mutation rate (which can also include rates of chromosome aberration production by UV), induction of oncogenic viruses by low UV doses, and increased malignant transformation of UV-damaged cells by oncogenic viruses. Since XP cells presumably only possess the repair system resembling recombination in bacteria, the strand breaks and strand exchanges involved in that system might provide loci for the integration of viruses. Ironically, with the precedents set by information we already have from *E. coli* and tumor virus work, all three of these alternatives may prove experimentally demonstrable, though none have yet been described for XP. XP may provide us with a tool for understanding some of the mechanisms that result in expression of altered genetic information in a cancer cell.

References

1. Aaronson, S.A. and Lytle, C.D. Decreased host cell reactivation of irradiated SV40 virus in xeroderma pigmentosum. Nature 228, 359 (1970).

2. Bootsma, D., Mulder, M.P., Pot, F. and Cohen, J.A. Different inherited levels of DNA repair replication in xeroderma pigmentosum cell strains after exposure to ultraviolet light. Mutation Res. 9, 507 (1970).

3. Cleaver, J.E. Defective repair replication of DNA in xeroderma pigmentosum. Nature 218, 652 (1968).

4. Cleaver, J.E. Xeroderma pigmentosum: a human disease in which an initial stage of DNA repair is defective. Proc. Nat. Acad. Sci. U.S.A. 63, 428 (1969).

5. Cleaver, J.E. DNA damage and repair in light-sensitive human skin disease. J. Invest. Derm. 54, 8 (1970).

6. Cleaver, J.E. DNA repair and radiation sensitivity in human (xeroderma pigmentosum) cells. Int. J. Radiat. Biol. 18, 557 (1970).

7. Cleaver, J.E. Repair of alkylation damage in ultraviolet-sensitive (xeroderma pigmentosum) human cells. Mutation Res. 12, 453 (1971).

8. Cleaver, J.E. Repair of damaged DNA in human and other eukaryotic cells. In Nucleic Acid Synthesis in Viral Infection, D.W. Ribbons, J.F. Woessner and J. Schultz, Eds., North-Holland Pub. Co., p. 87, 1971.

9. Epstein, J.H., Fukayama, K., Reed, W.B. and Epstein, W.L. Defect in DNA synthesis in skin of patients with xeroderma pigmentosum demonstrated in vivo. Science 168, 1477 (1970).

10. German, J. Bloom's syndrome, Fanconi's syndrome, ataxia telangiectesia, and xeroderma pigmentosum. In Proceedings Symposium on Biology of Skin, in press, 1972.

11. Jung, E.G. New form of molecular defect in xeroderma pigmentosum. Nature 228, 361 (1970).

12. Rabson, A.S., Tyrell, S.A. and Legallais, F.Y. Growth of ultraviolet-damaged herpes virus in xeroderma pigmentosum cells. Proc. Soc. Exptl. Biol. Med. 132, 802 (1969).

13. Rook, A., Wilkinson, D.S. and Ebling, F.J. Text-book of Dermatology, Vol. I. Oxford and Edinburgh, Blackwell, 1968, p. 62.

14. Setlow, R.B., Regan, J.D., German, J. and Carrier, W.L. Evidence that xeroderma pigmentosum cells do not perform the first step in the repair of ultraviolet damage to their DNA. Proc. Nat. Acad. Sci. U.S.A. 64, 1035 (1969).

15. Stich, H.G., San, R.H.C. and Kawazoe, Y. DNA repair synthesis in mammalian cells exposed to a series of oncogenic and non-oncogenic derivatives of 4-nitroquinoline oxide. Nature 229, 416 (1971).

16. Weerd-Kastelein, E.A., Keijzer, W. and Bootsma, D. Genetic heterogeneity of xeroderma pigmentosum demonstrated by somatic cell hybridization. Nature 238, 80 (1972).

CELL TRANSFORMATION BY POLYOMA VIRUS AND SV40

Walter Eckhart

The Salk Institute for Biological Studies
San Diego, California   92112

This lecture will be concerned with viral gene
functions and cell transformation. Several reviews
have been published recently that supply more extensive literature citations than will be included here
(5,13-15).

Transformation refers to the hereditary aquisi-
tion of altered growth properties by cells in culture.
The altered growth properties of transformed cells can
be assayed in several ways: generally speaking, transformed cells have altered morphology, high saturation
density, require lower amounts of serum for optimal
growth than normal cells, sometimes form colonies in
soft agar, and can form tumors when injected into
appropriate animals.

Transformation by RNA viruses is discussed in the
first lecture series. I shall discuss transformation
by the DNA tumor viruses, polyoma and SV40. Polyoma
virus and SV40 are small DNA viruses, having DNA with
a molecular weight of approximately 3×10^6, sufficient to code for the synthesis of 170,000 daltons of
protein, or about five proteins of average size.
These viruses are particularly useful for investigations of the role of viral genes in cell transformation because they code for such a small number of
proteins.

Several lines of evidence indicate that viral
genetic material persists and functions in transformed
cells. Virus specific RNA can be detected in trans-

formed cells, and DNA sequences homologous to viral
DNA are present, in some cases associated with cellular DNA by alkali stable bonds, suggesting covalent
linkage with the cellular DNA. In the case of SV40
transformed cells, infectious virus can often be res-
cued from the transformed cells by co-cultivation or
fusion with the cells susceptible to lytic infection.

Infection of cells by polyoma virus or SV40 can
lead either to a lytic reaction, with production of
infectious progeny virus and death of the host cell,
or to abortive infection, in which the virus growth
cycle is blocked at some stage before the production
of infectious progeny, and the host cell survives and
continues to grow. In the case of polyoma virus,
mouse cells usually give a lytic response to infection,
whereas hamster or rat cells usually give the abortive
type of response.

A general picture that emerges of the process of
transformation by polyoma virus or SV40 is that the
virus enters the host cell, becomes part of the hereditary material of the cell (in some cases by integration into the cellular DNA), and causes an alteration in cell growth regulation, either by making a
viral gene product that alters the host cell, or by
otherwise interfering in normal cellular regulatory
processes. In order to understand transformation in
detail, it would be desirable to know the products of
each of the viral genes, particularly the genes involved in transformation, and the state of the viral
DNA in the transformed cell, particularly with regard
to the regulation of viral gene expression.

In order to identify the viral gene products,
several kinds of viral mutants have been selected.
These mutants are listed in Table 1. Temperature-
sensitive (ts) mutants are selected on the basis of
their ability to form plaques at low (permissive)
temperature, but not at high (nonpermissive) temperature. Temperature-sensitive mutants can be used to
investigate the involvement of viral gene functions
in cell regulation by examining the properties of
cells infected or transformed by ts mutants at non-

permissive temperature, where the altered viral gene
function is inactive.

TABLE 1
POLYOMA VIRUS AND SV40 MUTANTS

1. Temperature sensitive
2. Host range
3. Hybrid viruses (Adeno-SV40)
4. Deletion (or other) defective

Host range mutants are a class of conditional
lethal mutants that are selected on the basis of their
ability to grow in transformed, superinfectable cells,
but not in untransformed cells (1). The rationale behind this selection is that if viral gene functions
are expressed in the transformed cell by the trans-
forming genome, these viral functions should be able
to allow the growth of mutants defective in the same
functions, whereas such mutants would not be able to
grow in untransformed cells, where the viral gene
functions cannot be supplied.

The adenovirus-SV40 hybrid viruses contain varying amounts of SV40 genetic material covalently linked
within an adenovirus genome (10). These viruses should
be very useful for physical mapping of the SV40 genome
by the technique of heteroduplex mapping. They may
also be used to investigate aspects of the control of
transcription and translation of viral messages in
infected cells.

Polyoma and SV40 virus stocks contain defective
particles, the concentration of which can be enriched
by passage of the virus stock at high multiplicities
of infection (17). These defective particles may
contain deletions or insertions of DNA, and would,
therefore, be expected to be mutated in the region of
the deletion or insertion. Such defective particles
could provide another source of mutants for the study
of viral gene functions. A problem that has not yet
been overcome is the difficulty in cloning such deletion or insertion mutants. Presumably this might be

accomplished by propagating the mutants on transformed, superinfectable cells to provide some missing
functions (as in the case of the host range mutants),
or by propagating them together with wild-type viruses
from which they could be separated on the basis of
their physical characteristics.

Before considering the results of experiments
using temperature-sensitive mutants of polyoma virus,
let us review some of the changes that take place in
cells infected by polyoma virus. These changes are
summarized in Table 2. There is an activation of
synthesis of cellular DNA and of the enzymes concerned
with DNA metabolism and a stimulation of cell movement.

TABLE 2
VIRUS INDUCED CHANGES IN POLYOMA
VIRUS INFECTED CELLS

1. Activation: cellular DNA synthesis
                 cellular enzyme synthesis
                 cell movement
2. T antigen (nuclear)
3. Transplantation antigen (cell surface)
4. Cell surface alteration (agglutinability)
5. Viral DNA and protein synthesis
6. Transformation: abortive
                     stable

Two new antigens appear: the T antigen is confined
to the nucleus, and is detected by immunofluorescence
or complement fixation; the transplantation antigen is
expressed in the cell surface, and is detected by
graft rejection by sensitized animals, or by cell
killing *in vitro*. Both antigens are virus specific;
that is, the antigens of polyoma virus infected cells
are different from the antigens of SV40 infected cells.
There is also an alteration of the cell surface, detected by enhanced agglutination of infected cells by
wheat germ agglutinin or Concanavalin A. Viral DNA
and protein synthesis take place in infected cells.
A certain fraction of infected cells become transformed.

Abortive transformation refers to the transient acquisition of some of the properties of transformed cells by infected cells, for example the ability to multiply in methyl cellulose suspension or in medium containing low amounts of serum. Stable transformation refers to the hereditary acquisition of transformed cell properties.

Temperature-sensitive mutants of polyoma virus have been isolated and characterized by genetic complementation tests and biochemical analysis (3,4,7). The mutants that have been studied so far can be placed into at least four groups, the properties of which are shown in Table 3. There are two late groups, containing mutants that are able to synthesize viral DNA at nonpermissive temperature, but not infectious virus particles. The two early groups contain mutants that are defective in viral DNA synthesis at nonpermissive temperature. The late mutants transform normally at nonpermissive temperature, indicating that the viral gene functions in which they are defective are not involved in transformation. Mutants in each of the two early groups show defects in transformation, and these will be discussed in more detail.

TABLE 3
PROPERTIES OF POLYOMA VIRUS
TEMPERATURE SENSITIVE MUTANTS

Function at nonper-missive temperature	Mutant Group			
	Late	Late	Early	Early
Viral DNA	+	+	−	−
Transformation	+	+	−	Temperature dependent
Cellular DNA	+	+	+	−
T Antigen (IF)	+	ND	−	ND

ND= not done

One of the early mutant groups, the ts–a group, contains mutants that are defective in viral DNA synthesis, and also in transformation, at the nonpermissive temperature. The requirement of the ts–a group function for transformation is a transient one, however, cells that are transformed at permissive temperature retain their transformed characteristics when grown at nonpermissive temperatures. Therefore, the ts–a gene function is required for initiation or stabilization of transformation, but not for maintenance of the state.

One can ask whether the requirement for the ts–a function in viral DNA synthesis is also a transient one, as would be the case, for example, if the ts–a function were required only for some initial event during the viral growth cycle. To test this, we have performed temperature shift experiments using ts–a infected cells shifted from permissive to nonpermissive temperature at various times during the virus growth cycle. The cells are labeled with tritiated thymidine after the shift to nonpermissive temperature, and synthesis of viral DNA is measured by incorporation of radioactive thymidine into DNA with the sedimentation characteristics of viral DNA. The results of such experiments show that viral DNA synthesis decays quickly in ts–a infected cells after a shift from permissive to nonpermissive temperature, the incorporation being less than 10% of the control value (in cells kept at permissive temperature) after 30 minutes. Wild-type infected cells continue to synthesize viral DNA at both temperatures. It can be concluded that the ts–a gene function is required continuously in order for viral DNA synthesis to take place. Further experiments may reveal at what stage in the replication process the ts–a function acts.

Together with M. Oxman and K. Takemoto, we have done experiments to test the ability of mutants in the ts–a group to synthesize polyoma T antigen detectable by immunofluorescence after infection of mouse embryo cells (11). The results of these experiments show that three early mutants, like ts–a, do not synthesize

T antigen detectable by immunofluorescence at nonpermissive temperature, whereas one late mutant does so normally at nonpermissive temperature. The inability of the early mutants to synthesize T antigen is not a consequence of their inability to synthesize viral DNA, because T antigen is produced by wild-type polyoma in the presence of inhibitors of DNA synthesis. At present it is not possible to decide whether the ts-a gene is the structural gene for T antigen, or whether the ts-a gene product is required somehow for synthesis or detection of T antigen in the infected cells.

Although the ts-a function is required for viral DNA synthesis, it is not required for the induction of cellular DNA synthesis (8). From the T antigen experiments it follows that the production of T antigen detectable by immunofluorescence is not required for induction of cellular DNA synthesis, but may be required for viral DNA synthesis.

What could the ts-a function be? The observations that the ts-a function is required continuously for viral DNA synthesis, and that it is required for initiation or stabilization of transformation, have led to supposition that it may be an enzyme involved in DNA replication and recombination, perhaps a "nicking" enzyme. More definitive evidence may come from a closer analysis of the process of viral DNA replication, or from an analysis of enzymes in ts-a infected cells.

The second early mutant group contains a single mutant, ts3. The ts3 function is required for the expression of several virus mediated effects in the infected cells: induction of host DNA synthesis, viral DNA synthesis, and surface alteration as monitored by agglutination by wheat germ agglutinin or Concanavalin A. In cells transformed by ts3, certain aspects of the transformed phenotype are temperature dependent (6). Surface alteration, measured by agglutination, and density-dependent inhibition of DNA synthesis are both dependent upon temperature. The ts3 transformed cells behave like normal cells in these parameters when grown at nonpermissive temperature, but behave like transformed cells when grown at permissive temperature. This result implies that the ts3 gene function is required for maintenance of certain properties of transformed cells. Other properties, like the ability to grow in agar, are not temperature dependent in ts3 transformed cells. Either growth in agar is not dependent upon the ts3 gene product, or the ts3 gene product is required in lower amounts for growth in agar than for the expression of other transformed cell properties.

How could the ts3 function act? It could act directly on infected or transformed cells, by changing some chemical groups in the cell surface, for example. Alternatively, it could act indirectly, by altering the expression of viral or cellular genes in the infected or transformed cell. The pleiotropic effects of the mutation in infected cells suggest that the ts3 gene function may play a regulatory role.

The behavior of ts3 transformed cells implies that at least one viral gene product is required in order to maintain some properties of transformed cells. Until the mechanism of action of the gene product is known, however, it is not possible to say whether the viral gene function causes transformation directly, or acts by derepressing host cell genes that in turn are responsible for the alterations in cell growth regulation.

The results of exepriments with host range mutants support the interpretation that cell surface alterations are important in cell growth regulation (2). Four host range mutants of polyoma virus have been isolated. All four are defective in transformation, in agreement with the rationale behind the selection procedure, discussed earlier. The host range mutants are also defective in producing the surface alteration detected by agglutination after infection, although they do induce cellular DNA synthesis. The host range mutants are weakly temperature-sensitive, and it may be possible to take advantage of this fact to test whether the gene product in which they are defective is required to maintain aspects of the transformed cell phenotype, as has been done with the ts3 mutant.

Both contact between cells, and requirement for growth factors present in serum, appear to influence the growth regulation of cells in culture. At present it is difficult to assess the relative importance of contact *vs.* serum factors, because it is possible that sparse cells are more sensitive to the action of serum factors, or have lower requirements for serum factors, that crowded cells. The ts3 gene function seems to affect contact mediated effects, rather than serum requirements in transformed cells. Whether this means that the two kinds of effects can be separated, or whether their expression simply requires different amounts of the viral gene product, remains to be determined.

In the selection of temperature-sensitive mutants, it would be desirable to know whether there are viral functions that are required for transformation, but not for lytic growth of the virus. Such gene functions would not be detected by the selection procedures that depends upon differential lytic growth at two temperatures. We have tried to address this question by the following experiment: wild-type polyoma virus is inactivated highly with nitrous acid, and survivors are assayed by plaque assay. From a virus stock that has been inactivated to a survival of about 10^{-5}, survivors that are able to form plaques are picked and repurified by successive plaque isolation. If there is a gene that is required for transformation, but not for lytic infection, this gene should have been damaged by the nitrous acid treatment, and some of the survivors should not transform. Of 12 survivors assayed for ability to transform, all 12 were able to transform normally, implying that there is no viral gene required for transformation that is not required for lytic infection in this system. Unfortunately this conclusion is not a firm one, because we have no independent measurement of how much of the nitrous acid inactivation is caused by inactivation of gene function, rather than, for example, inactivation of ability of the genome to replicate because of structural damage. At this level of inactivation, about 1% of the survivors are temperature-sensitive mutants, so some alterations that affect gene function must occur, but until the nature of the damage can be characterized more thoroughly, the existence of viral genes that affect transformation, but are not necessary for lytic growth, should not be ruled out.

How much of the coding capacity of the viral genome is devoted to making proteins of the virion? Virion proteins have been examined by electrophoresis in SDS-polyacrylamide gels (9,12). The major structural protein of the virion, which comprises about 70% of the total virion protein, has a molecular weight of about 45,000. There are two proteins with molecular weights of 30-35,000, and 18-23,000 respectively, and three small proteins of molecular weight 10-15,000. The three small proteins may be coded for by the cell, because they are found to be enriched, relative to the other proteins, for amino acids derived from cells labeled prior to infection. Definitive evidence for viral coded proteins in the virion would come from experiments showing that mutants of the virus contain proteins with altered amino acid sequences. Until this, or some other definitive experiment, is done, it is not possible to say with certainty that all three larger proteins are virus coded. If one assumes that they are coded for by the virus, approximately half of the coding capacity of the virus would be devoted to the synthesis of virion proteins.

The problem of associating viral gene functions with identifiable proteins is being attacked in two ways by several laboratories. First, the proteins of infected cells are analyzed by sensitive polyacrylamide gel electrophoresis to determine whether new proteins appear after infection, or whether some proteins already present before infection are modified. This kind of experiment is technically difficult because infection by polyoma virus does not result in a shutoff of host protein synthesis, as is the case with some lytic animal viruses. Second, efforts are being made to synthesize proteins *in vitro*, using protein synthesizing systems derived from *E. coli*. These experiments have given some encouraging results,

but the uncertainties of the specificity of action of
the RNA polymerase and translation machinery of the
system, when presented with mammalian virus DNA, make
it difficult to interpret the results.

Recently there has been speculation about the
possibility of integration of viral DNA with cellular
DNA during lytic infection. Virus specific sequences
are found in the high molecular weight heterogeneous
RNA in the nuclei of infected cells, and it is possible
that single transcripts may contain both viral and
cellular sequences. Several laboratories are looking
for direct physical evidence of integration during
lytic infection.

One striking feature of the DNA tumor viruses is
their long latent period. It takes eight to twelve
hours after lytic infection before virus specific
proteins are detected in infected cultures, and about
18 hours before viral DNA synthesis begins. The
length of the latent period depends upon the multiplicity of infection. The long latent period suggests
that there may be a stage in the cell cycle that is
required for part of the infection by polyoma virus
or SV40, and that infected cells must reach this
stage before the infecting virus is able to replicate.

Regulation of viral gene expression in transformed
cells is important for expression of the transformed
phenotype. For this reason, many groups have attacked
the problem of regulation of viral gene expression by
studying the transcription of viral DNA in transformed
cells. In at least some cases, only part of the viral
genome is transcribed in transformed cells. Although
selective breakdown of certain RNA sequences cannot be
ruled out, the most attractive interpretation of this
result is that there is regulation of viral gene expression at the level of transcription in these cell
lines.

Studies of the size of virus-specific RNA in
transformed cells have shown that there are virus-
specific sequences in large RNA molecules in the
nucleus. Some of these molecules are larger than a
single transcript of the viral DNA. The virus specific

sequences in the cytoplasm are present in smaller RNA molecules, implying that some processing step occurs between transcription in the nucleus and association with ribosomes in the cytoplasm. There is evidence that the virus specific RNAs in the nucleus are transcribed into molecules that also contain cellular sequences (16). Therefore, regulation of transcription may be accomplished by virtue of the association of viral DNA with cellular DNA, which results in the utilization of new promoter or terminator sites for transcription.

The transformed phenotype is most likely the result of the interaction of viral and cellular functions. Revertants of virus-transformed cells can be selected that have lost some or all of the growth characteristics of transformed cells, while still containing a functional viral genome. Therefore, the presence of a functioning viral genome is not sufficient to cause transformation, or, if it is sufficient, its effect can be overcome by an appropriate combination of cellular gene functions.

To summarize: two gene functions of polyoma virus are involved in cell transformation. One function is required for viral DNA synthesis, and for initiation or stabilization of transformation, but not for maintenance of the transformed phenotype. The other function is required for the expression of several virus mediated changes in the infected cell early during lytic infection, and is required continuously for the maintenance of cell surface properties and loss of contact inhibition of DNA synthesis characteristic of transformed cells. Future work will be aimed at characterizing these viral gene functions more precisely in order to determine how they act to influence transformation, and at trying to understand the relationships between cell surface properties, control of DNA synthesis, and growth regulation that seem to be important features of the regulatory systems of animal cells.

References

1. Benjamin, T.L. Host range mutants of polyoma virus. Proc. Nat. Acad. Sci. U.S.A. 67, 394 (1970).

2. Benjamin, T.L., and Burger, M.M. Absence of a cell membrane alteration function in non-transforming mutants of polyoma virus. Proc. Nat. Acad. Sci. U.S.A. 67, 929 (1970).

3. di Mayorca, G., Callender, J., Marin, G., and Giordano, R. Temperature-semsitive mutants of polyoma virus. Virology 38, 126 (1969).

4. Eckhart, W. Complementation and transformation by temperature sensitive mutants of polyoma virus. Virology 38, 120 (1969).

5. Eckhart, W. Oncogenic viruses. Ann. Rev. Biochem. 41, 503 (1972).

6. Eckhart, W., Dulbecco, R., and Burger, M. Temperature dependent surface changes in cells infected or transformed by a thermosensitive mutant of polyoma virus. Proc. Nat. Acad. Sci. U.S.A. 68 283 (1971).

7. Fried, M. Cell transformation ability of a temperature sensitive mutant of polyoma virus. Proc. Nat. Acad. Sci. U.S.A. 53, 486 (1965).

8. Fried, M. Characterization of a temperature sensitive mutant of polyoma virus. Virology 40, 605 (1970).

9. Hirt, B., and Gesteland, R.F. Characterization of the proteins of SV40 and polyoma virus. In Biology of Oncogenic Viruses, L. Silvestri (ed.), p. 98, 1971.

10. Lewis, A.M., Levin, M.J., Wiese, W.H., Crimpacker, C.S., and Henry, P.H. A nondefective (competent) adenovirus-SV40 hybrid isolated from the AD2-SV40 hybrid population. Proc. Nat. Acad. Sci. U.S.A. 63, 1128 (1969).

11. Oxman, M., Takemoto, K., and Eckhart, W. Polyoma T antigen synthesis by temperature sensitive mutants of polyoma, submitted for publication.

12. Roblin, R., Harle, E., Dulbecco, R. Polyoma virus proteins. _Virology_ 45, 555 (1971).
13. Sambrook, J. Transformation by polyoma virus and SV40. _Adv. Cancer Res._, in press.
14. Silvestri, L., Ed. _The Biology of Oncogenic Viruses_. North-Holland, Amsterdam, 1971.
15. Tooze, J., Ed. _The Molecular Biology of Animal Tumor Viruses_. Cold Spring Harbor, New York, in press.
16. Wall, R., and DArnell, J.E. Presence of cell and virus specific sequences in the same molecules of nuclear RNA from virus transformed cells. _Nature New Biol._ 232, 73 (1971).
17. Yoshiiki, K. Studies on DNA from low-density particles of SV40. _Virology_ 34, 391 (1968).

IMMUNO-GENETICS IN THE STUDY OF CELL SURFACES: SOME IMPLICATIONS FOR MORPHOGENESIS AND CANCER

Edward A. Boyse

Sloan-Kettering Institute for Cancer Research
New York, New York 10021

The subject of my presentation is the antigenic structure of cell surfaces. To be more precise I shall be describing some of the ways in which immuno-genetics has been used to study the constitution of cell surfaces.

I think I can indicate, at the outset, something about the relevance of this to cancer in a very few words. It is obvious that the genome of the fertilized ovum, or zygote, of a metazoan carries instructions for a program of great complexity that will result in the controlled deployment of a vast number of accurately diversified progeny cells to produce the complete organism, - the process known as *morphogenesis*. It is widely believed that one essential component of morphogenesis is the ability of cells to recognize one another and so to participate in orderly assemblies, which means in effect that the genome's instructions for morphogenesis are largely implemented by the cell surface. Therefore in finding out more about how the surface of each differentiated cell is genetically specified, and about how the resultant gene products are put together to form the cell surface, we are clearly working on a problem of central importance in biology.

Three features of cancer particularly show it to be a disorder of morphogenesis or morphostasis. First, to a greater or lesser extent, cancer cells fail to organize themselves into normal biological patterns but instead exhibit a more or less chaotic histology. Sec- one, they fail to form relevant relationships with adjoining normal cells, so that they invade normal tissues. Third, they settle and grow in incongruous sites (metastasis).

Thus, unless we are greatly mistaken in our belief that the cell surface is a medium through which the genome directs morphogenesis, we must believe that the full account of cancer, when it comes to be written, will involve understanding of how systems of recognition are built into the cell surface as well as of how the mechanism breaks down in cancer. In fact it is virtually axiomatic that the systematic study of normal cell surfaces may, in the long run, be at least as relevant to understanding the biology of cancer as is the study of tumor antigens on the cell surface. Considering the great importance which we therefore attach to the constitution of the cell surface in the social organization of cells, it is intimidating to realize how little we know about it. So our initial questions must be very simple ones, such as: What set of genes and gene products go into the making of each particular cell surface? What rules of assembly may the different molecular constituents of the cell surface obey?

The tools which seem most adequate to this task at the present time are those of immunogenetics. This is because antigenicity provides a relatively simple and commonly feasible label for identifying gene products regardless of their function. Antigens, in other words, are highly convenient labels for distinguishing one element of the cell surface from another. In most of the contexts I shall mention, the fact that a given constitutent of the cell surface can be recognized as an antigen is relevant only in so far as the respective antibody can be used as a label.

Adequate serological methods for studying the surfaces of nucleated cells have come into use only in recent years, so I believe the best way for me to present you with a brief review of the field is to do so chronologically. Perhaps the subject is still young enough to made the chronological approach not only feasible but perhaps also most apt for outlining the field for non-immunologists.

I shall spend this discussion describing how a number of important systems were first revealed and analyzed, and will try to keep this as simple as possible. In the second part, I shall discuss several goals that may be approached by working with these systems.

* * * * * * * *

The beginning of definitive serological work with nucleated cells in the mouse was in 1956, the year in which Gorer (10) devised the cytotoxicity test (Figure 1) for detecting antigens on cell surfaces. At that time much was known about blood groups in several species, and much could be inferred from studies of histocompatibility antigens *in vivo*, but no well-defined systems of serologically demonstrable antigens on viable nucleated cells were known. Gorer's cytotoxicity test opened new possibilities, and it remains today the mainstay for serological analysis of new antigenic systems on nucleated cells.

CYTOTOXICITY TEST

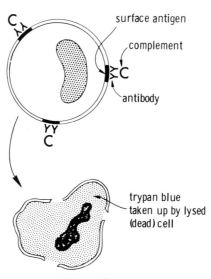

Fig. 1

The basis of Gorer's test is that nucleated cells
are lysed when exposed, in the presence of complement,
to antibody against any of their surface components.
The cell surface is actually perforated, so that the
contents leak out, and large external molecules can
enter. So the assay for cytotoxic antibody can be
based on release of radioactivity from cells previously
labeled with ^{51}Cr, or more simply on the uptake of the
dye trypan blue, which living cells exclude. The latter was used by Gorer, and is the simplest criterion
of a positive result. After the cells have been incu-
bated with antibody and complement for half-an-hour,
trypan blue is added, and the result is determined by
counting live (unstained) and dead (trypan-blue-stained)
cells in a counting chamber. Actually the dead cells
are morphologically distinguishable from the living
cells, but the addition of trypan blue makes reading
much easier. The test has undergone many improvements
and refinements, mainly in the way in which serum complement is used in the test, and these are mainly responsible for the successful description of new systems.
It is now an altogether much more sentitive method than
when it first came into use in 1956.

As so many things seem to hinge on the constitution of the cell surface, it is obvious that in attempt-
ing to review the field rather generally, I shall touch
on a number of different topics, and that I can comment
on each of them only briefly.

* * * * * * * *

Gorer devised the cytotoxicity test to demonstrate
H-2 antigens on nucleated cells of the mouse (Figure 2).
H-2 was already known to be the major histocompatibility
locus of the mouse, but until that time its serological
analysis had depended entirely on red cell typing, just
like any of the human blood groups, for example. All
mouse cells carry H-2 antigens on their surfaces. Different mice carry different H-2 alleles and so have
different H-2 antigens. The cytotoxicity test can be
used to demonstrate H-2 on thymocytes, lymphocytes,

spleen cells, bone marrow cells, ascites tumors and any other cells that are freely obtainable in viable suspension. Other tissues are shown to carry H-2 by their capacity to absorb H-2 antibody specifically from H-2 antisera. (For an account of the H-2 system see 18.)

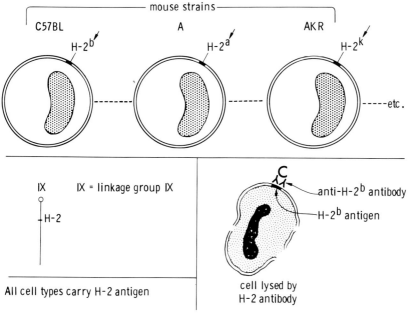

H-2 SYSTEM

Major histocompatibility antigens of mice

Fig. 2

One comment on this figure is important to understanding much of what I shall have to say later. Because different mouse strains carry different H-2 genes or alleles, they can be immunized, one against the other, to produce different H-2 antisera, and so the entire system can be analyzed serologically with antibodies produced in the same species, the mouse. Now the general aim of most of the work I shall describe is to study the constitution of cell surfaces in terms of the gene products of which they are composed and of

61

how these are organized. My point is that in order to do this we are usually forced to limit attention to components like H-2 which are variable throughout the species, *i.e.*, where the determinant genes are polymorphic and antisera can be made by immunizing one mouse strain against another. An antiserum prepared against mouse cells in the rabbit for example will recognize antigens present on all mouse cells (*e.g.*, MSLA: "Mouse Specific Lymphocyte Antigen," in Figure 11 below) but such antibodies are of little value in analyzing the cell surface, for it is not possible to make crosses to test segregating populations and so find out how many antigens are being recognized, what genes are involved, and where the genes are. Thus, in general, one cannot find out with such an antiserum which or how many components of the cell surface such antisera may be reacting with. For the most part therefore we must deal with allo-antisera, *i.e.*, antibodies produced by immunizing one inbred strain of mouse against another. When such an antiserum gives a positive test in a given system, hopefully the reaction can be traced to a single gene by conventional segregation tests, the locus of the gene can be assigned to a particular chromosome by linkage tests (as H-2 has been located in Linkage Group IX), and one would now, for example, be justified in trying to isolate and characterize the gene product on which the newly recognized antigen is situated.

* * * * * * * *

In 1965 a second cell surface antigen called Gross Cell Surface Antigen or GCSA came to light during some early studies on the surface antigens of leukemia cells (12).

AKR is a strain of mouse that has a very high incidence of leukemia due to natural life-long infection with the murine leukemia virus (MLV) discovered by Gross. Cells producing MLV, whether they have undergone leukemic transformation or not, are not killed, but continue to produce virus indefinitely by budding from the cell surface. Gross observed that some strains of mice are susceptible to leukemia-induction by this virus, and others resistant. Strain C57BL is one of the most resistant, although an occasiona leukemia can be induced by inoculating large amounts of virus into newborn recipients. Suspecting that leukemia cells induced by MLV might carry antigen related to MLV, and that at least part of the resistance of C57BL mice might be due to an ability to respond immunologically to this antigen, we set up the immunization shown diagramatically in Figure 3, in which C57BL mice received repeated inoculations of increasing numbers of AKR lymphoid cells or leukemia cells, both of which produce

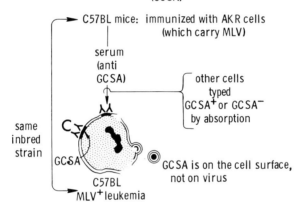

GROSS CELL SURFACE ANTIGEN
(GCSA)

GCSA is found on all MLV$^+$ (wild-type) leukemias

Fig. 3

MLV. The resulting antiserum must contain H-2 antibodies as well as antibodies to other normal tissue antigens for which C57BL and AKR differ, in addition to the hypothetical leukemia-specific antibody. This difficulty is circumvented by testing the C57BL antiserum on a leukemia induced by Gross leukemia virus in the C57BL strain itself. Since the mice producing the antiserum are syngeneic with the leukemic test cells, any cytotoxic reaction must be specific for leukemia antigen. As shown here, this immunization does produce cytotoxic antibody of relatively high titer against Gross leukemia cells. We called the antigen recognized Gross Cell Surface Antigen or GCSA. The GCSA system can be analyzed further by absorption. In other word,, any cells can now be typed for GCSA by testing whether they do or do not remove cytotoxic activity against the standard C57BL Gross leukemia cells as indicated here.

Analyzing a new system by absorption in this way is a valuable method, and sometimes the only feasible one. Although one might expect GCSA to be an antigen of the leukemia virus coat, Aoki (1) has shown, by immuno-ferritin labeling, that it is not. It is found at cell surface sites where leukemia virus is not budding. Figure 4 gives the essentials of the GCSA system: In strains like AKR that have a high incidence of leukemia, the lymphoid organs are GCSA$^+$ throughout life, as might be expected from the fact that they are producing leukemia virus. Lymphoid tissues of strains with a low incidence of leukemia, like C57BL, are characteristically GCSA$^-$. On the other hand, in at least most strains of mice there occur some leukemias which are GCSA$^+$. This did not seem unduly surprising, for it appeared reasonable that the virus should occasionally produce leukemias in mice that are not overt virus carriers, as well as in the high-incidence carrier strains like AKR.

GCSA

	lymphoid cells	MLV$^+$ leukemias (spontaneous or induced)
AKR*	+	+
C57BL*	−	+

*representative mouse strains

Questions: 1) why are immunized mice not resistant to transplants?
2) inheritance?

Fig. 4

With the recognition of GCSA we have a second class of cell surface antigens, this time apparently specified by a virus, in contrast to normal allo-antigens represented by H-2. It is noteworthy, also, that the antigen in this case is not ubiquitous on mouse cells but is generally restricted to lymphoid tissue.

We were puzzled to find that C57BL mice immunized with AKR tissues, and producing high titers of cytotoxic GCSA antibody, were not highly resistant to transplants of the C57BL Gross leukemia. Why is immunization against GCSA of such little value in protecting mice against $GCSA^+$ transplanted leukemias, when it is clear there has been a substantial immune response in the form of GCSA antibody? We shall return to this paradox later when I discuss antigenic modulation.

As there are both $GCSA^+$ and $GCSA^-$ strains of mice, it is possible to perform conventional genetic tests to establish the mode of inheritance. We did not study this intensively at first, mainly for the reason that it seemed unreasonable to expect Mendelian inheritance of an antigen that not only seemed to be specified by a virus but also appeared sporadically on leukemia cells of any strain of mice. In retrospect it is likely that the question should have been pressed a lot harder, as we shall see.

* * * * * * * *

The next antigenic system that came to light in our studies was the TL system of antigens (reviewed in 7), and this was discovered with a similar immunization schedule (Figure 5) to that described before. Having in mind that the leukemias occurring in low-incidence strains of mice are frequently $GCSA^-$, we set out to investigate whether these leukemias might be carrying a different antigen, possibly the product of a second leukemia virus of a different antigenic type.

C57BL mice were again used for immunization, but this time the immunizing cells came from a $GCSA^-$ leukemia occurring in the A strain, which is not an overt carrier of leukemia virus. As before, the antiserum

THYMUS-LEUKEMIA ANTIGEN
(TL)

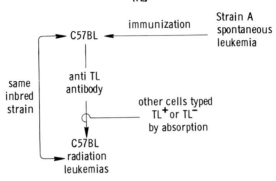

Fig. 5

was tested on leukemias arising in the strain producing
the antiserum, *i.e.*, C57BL. This time we needed a
C57BL leukemia not induced obviously by leukemia virus.
Fortunately, C57BL mice are highly sensitive to induction of leukemia by irradiation. So we used these
leukemias, which are usually *not* GCSA$^+$, as the source
of test cells. Once again a highly cytotoxic antiserum was obtained, and the new system was analyzed by
absorption. It turned out that this antigen also was
represented on normal cells of some mouse strains, but
in this case only on thymocytes. Having ascertained
that it was confined exclusively to thymocytes and
leukemia cells we named it TL (Thymus-Leukemia) antigen.
Just as mouse strains may be classed as GCSA$^+$ or GCSA$^-$
according to whether their lymphoid cells carry GCSA,
so mouse strains can be classified as TL$^+$ or TL$^-$ according to whether or not their thymocytes carry TL
antigen (Figure 6). And as in the case of GCSA, TL
antigens may appear on leukemias of all mouse strains,
whether the strain is TL$^-$ or TL$^+$. This is a striking
resemblance between the GCSA and TL systems, but the
notable difference is that no virus of any kind has so
far been identified in association with TL$^+$ thymocytes
or leukemia cells. We were therefore particularly
alert to the possibility that we might be looking at

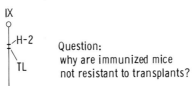

TL ANTIGENS

	thymocytes	leukemias**
A*	+	+
C57BL*	—	⊞

* representative mouse strains
** in every strain <u>some</u> leukemias are TL⁻

IX

H-2

TL

Question:
why are immunized mice
not resistant to transplants?

Fig. 6

an antigen specified by the genome of the cell rather than by a virus, despite the fact that TL antigen may appear on leukemia cells of all mouse strains, regardless of the TL type of the host. Inheritance was tested by crossing TL⁻ mice with TL⁺ mice, and obtaining backcross populations of mice whose thymocytes were typed TL⁺ or TL⁻. This revealed that thymic TL antigen is transmitted as a single Mendelian character, like other cell surface allo-antigens such as H-2. Linkage tests then showed that the responsible gene is located in linkage group IX of the mouse genome, quite close to H-2.

   To summarize, some strains of mice have TL⁻ thymocytes but are nevertheless carrying the respective TL gene, and this may become de-repressed in leukemia cells.

   It is far from clear how one should classify the TL antigens, of which four are now known, for there is an obvious parallel with GCSA in the sporadic occurrence of antigen in leukemias of all strains, and yet their inheritance on thymocytes is strictly Mendelian like normal allo-antigens such as H-2.

   Another parallel with GCSA is that mice immunized against TL and producing high titers of TL antibody have scarcely, if any, resistance to transplants of TL⁺ leukemias of the same inbred strain.

This paradox was partly explained when it was found that the effect of TL antibody on TL^+ cells is to delete TL antigen from the cell surface for as long as antibody is present, after which the antigen is fully expressed once more (Figure 7). By studying this phenomenon *in vitro*, exposing TL^+ cells to TL antibody in the absence of complement, it was ascertained that the change in phenotype from TL^+ to TL^-, which we now call *antigenic modulation*, is an adaptive one affecting TL^+ cells within minutes of exposure to TL antibody. Aoki (unpublished) has since found a similar loss of GCSA from Gross leukemia cells passed in immunized mice, and so it seems likely that antigenic modulation is the reason why immunization against GCSA also is ineffective in protecting mice from transplants of $GCSA^+$ leukemia cells.

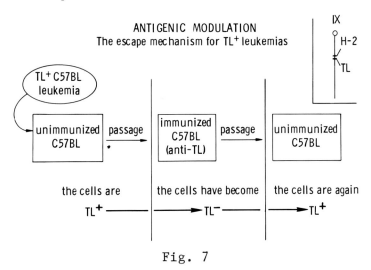

ANTIGENIC MODULATION
The escape mechanism for TL^+ leukemias

Fig. 7

To avoid giving the wrong impression, I must point out that immunity is not wholly ineffective against leukemias caused by wild-type MLV. For example, passive immunization of mice with antiserum produced in rats, which I shall describe in a moment, is highly effective in protecting mice against transplanted syngeneic Gross leukemia cells. What I said about modu-

lation in the Gross system is intended to apply spe-
cially to the antigen GCSA; rat antiserum contains'
antibodies to numerous other leukemia-related antigens
(see below).

To continue with the catalog of antigenic systems
now known on lymphoid cells - as I said earlier, the
use of absorption as a method of analyzing new systems
is valuable and often imperative, because of the presence of contaminating antibodies formed as a consequence of immunization with foreign cells. We were
aware, however, that some of these unidentified contaminating antibodies themselves were of interest,
particularly several that reacted preferentially with
the *thymocytes* of the strain providing the immunizing
tissue, as indeed TL antisera do. So once the GCSA
and TL systems were relatively well-defined we began
to analyze several of these anti-leukemia sera further to find out more about these anti-thymocyte antibodies. We also set up a series of planned immuniza-
tions with thymocytes, using donors and recipients of
the same H-2 type, to see whether further analyzable
systems could be unearthed.

The common type of lymphoid leukemia in the mouse
is a derivate of the thymocyte, or more strictly of
that lineage of cells which originate in bone marrow,
mature in the thymus, and migrate to lymphoid tissue
as what are now known as T lymphocytes. Consequently,
leukemias generally carry the surface antigens that
are characteristic of thymocytes. For this reason
thymocytes or leukemia cells can often be used inter-
changeably to produce antisera of the type required
to identify thymocyte antigens like TL. At about this
point in our studies, Reif in Boston reported a system of antigens which he called θ, and which were
recognized by immunizing one mouse strain with the
thymocytes of another (Figure 8). The thymocytes of
all strains of mice carried either of two alternative
θ antigens. Our own program turned up at least three
more such systems, called the Ly series, in which the
antigens identified were confined to T lymphocytes and
their precursors, the thymocytes. Several more Ly systems are in the process of being analyzed, but it seems

69

that there may be a large number of them and one doubts
whether it will be feasible to analyze them all, because of the large investment in time and animals that
is required for detailed description of each one of
them. In each case the T lymphocytes of every mouse
bear one or the other of two alternative antigens specified by alternative alleles at the relevant locus.
In each of the three cases listed here, the location
of the respective genes has been identified by linkage
tests. θ differs from the Ly group in that θ antigens
are expressed on brain and epidermal cells as well as
on T lymphocytes.

CELL-SURFACE DIFFERENTIATION ALLO-ANTIGENS OF THYMOCYTE/T-CELLS*

system	locus in linkage group	all mice express	antigen found on:		
			thymocytes	T-lymphocytes	other cells
θ	II	θ-AKR or θ-C3H	++	+	brain & skin
Ly-A	XII	Ly-A.1 or Ly-A.2	++	+	none
Ly-B,C	XI	Ly-B.1 or Ly-B.2 and	++	+	none
		Ly-C.1 or Ly-C.2	++	+	none

* excluding TL and other systems in which apparently no antigen is expressed
in some mouse strains.

Fig. 8

Although the θ/Ly antigens, like GCSA and TL, are
primarily lymphoid antigens, they are distinguished
from them by the fact that every mouse carries one or
the other alternative antigen, whereas in the case of
GCSA and TL, the difference between one mouse and
another consists in the presence or absence of the
respective antigen. This is no doubt associated with
the fact that both GCSA and TL antigens frequently
appear on leukemias of strains that normally do not
express them, signifying that normal mice of GCSA⁻ or
TL⁻ strains are carrying the relevant genes but not

expressing them (except in the event of leukemia) -,
whereas in the θ and Ly systems all mice are positive
for one or the other alternative antigen, and consequently we do not see or expect to see the anomalous
expression on leukemia cells that characterizes the
GCSA and TL systems. Although this θ/Ly group of antigens seems at first sight to take us rather far from
the subject of cancer, it may help to provide some insights into differentiation and morphogenesis, as I
shall discuss later (for review of these systems see
7).

* * * * * * * *

The last of the major systems I shall describe is
called G_{IX} (19), for reasons which will become clear.
It really belongs with the GCSA and TL class of antigens, and it comes last on my list only because I have
been taking the systems in the order in which they
were discovered. Anti-G_{IX} serum is obtained in the
following manner (Figure 9): Newborn rats are highly
susceptible to induction of leukemia by MLV from the
mouse, but the induced leukemias are so highly antigenic that they are commonly rejected when transplanted
to adult recipients, undoubtedly because the rat responds to a wider spectrum of virus-leukemia antigens
than the mouse. Consequently the serum of adult inbred rats that have rejected transplants of such leukemias induced in the same inbred rat strain is a rich
source of antibodies against viral components and
other antigens of MLV-infected cells. In addition,
such antiserum is cytotoxic for the thymocytes of several mouse strains that are not overt carriers of leukemia virus, and lack GCSA and all other recognized
leukemia virus antigens. This is a typical case for
analysis by absorption, using as test cells thymocytes
from a strain that has no GCSA antigen and is not
producing Gross virus (Figure 9). As in the GCSA and
TL systems, this set-up renders the serological test
specific for the newly recognized antigen. Bear in
mind that the rat has formed G_{IX} antibody in response
to G_{IX} antigen induced in the rat cells by mouse
leukemia virus; therefore the antigen must be coded

71

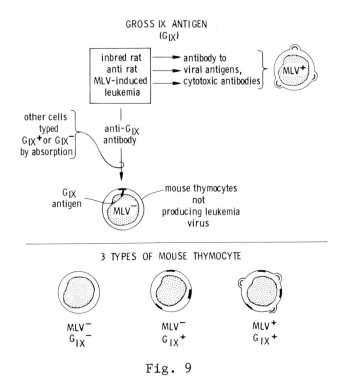

Fig. 9

by mouse leukemia virus itself, unless the virus has de-repressed a rat gene (shared by the mouse) which in turn produces the antigen. Using this absorption system the thymocytes of individual mice can be typed as positive or negative for this new antigen, which permits segregation analysis; this shows that inheritance of G_{IX} in normal mice is Mendelian. Actually *two* genes are required for expression of G_{IX} on thymocytes. One of these is in Linkage Group IX, like H-2 and TL, hence the designation G_{IX} (Gross IX) for the antigen. The location of the second gene is not yet certain.

When we turn to the typing of leukemias for G_{IX} antigen (Figure 10), we find the same familiar situation as was found in the GCSA and TL systems, namely that G_{IX} antigen is expressed on all leukemia cells

G_{IX} ANTIGEN

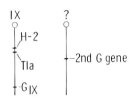

	thymocytes	MLV$^+$ leukemia cells
DBA/2^a	+	+
C57BL^a	—	+

^{a}representative mouse strains

Fig. 10

that carry MLV in all mouse strains regardless of whether the strain in which the leukemia arose does or does not carry G_{IX} antigen on its thymocytes.

* * * * * * * *

That completes the main inventory (Figure 11) of presently recognized antigen systems that occur on normal and malignant lymphoid cells. This is the basic information we have on the antigenic structures of these cells, and I would like to give a broad out-line in the rest of my discussion of what we think their their implications may be and what major problems they seem to present us with at the moment.

* * * * * * * *

Let us begin by asking some questions about the two systems that have something in common, G_{IX} and TL, and are in some way connected with leukemogenesis and/or leukemia virus. GCSA will not be considered, although it belongs here, because its inheritance has not strictly

73

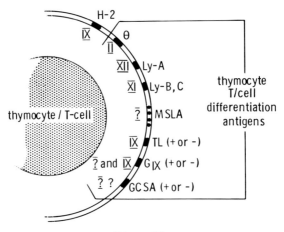

Fig. 11

been shown to be Mendelian, whereas TL and G_{IX} have been shown to be so inherited in normal mice. With regard to G_{IX}, we have seen that some mouse strains express G_{IX} on their thymocytes and others do not, whereas on leukemia cells G_{IX} does not obey the same rules, but may appear on leukemias of any strain (Figure 12).

	thymocytes	MLV+ leukemia cells
G_{IX}^+ mouse strains	G_{IX}^+	G_{IX}^+
G_{IX}^- mouse strains	G_{IX}^-	$\boxed{G_{IX}^+}$

Fig. 12: Anomalous appearance of G_{IX} antigen on MLV+ cells of G_{IX}^- mice.

On present evidence the appearance of G_{IX} antigen on leukemias of G_{IX}^- mouse strains results from activation of repressed leukemia virus, which according to prevailing opinion may be present in some form in all mice. G_{IX} antigen is probably not a structural component of the virus itself, so it is particularly difficult to decide whether it is coded by the MLV genome itself or by the cellular genome at the instigation of the virus. The former seems more likely from the fact that MLV induces the production of G_{IX} antigen in rat cells (see discussion in (19)).

In either event, one of the more important and reasonable hypotheses to consider, and if possible test, is that a leukemia virus genome is integrated at the G_{IX} locus in linkage group IX, exhibiting partial expression in the form of G_{IX} antigen in certain strains of mice. The situation with regard to anomalous expression of antigen in leukemias is similar for TL (Figure 13). These antigens also show Mendelian in-

	thymocytes	leukemia cells (often)
TL^+ mouse strains	TL^+	TL^+
TL^- mouse strains	TL^-	$\boxed{TL^+}$

Fig. 13: Anomalous appearance of TL antigens on leukemias of TL^- mice.

heritance in normal mice but appear in some leukemias of all strain of mice, whether the host is TL^- or TL^+. The outstanding difference is that, in this case, there is no evidence that the shift in phenotype from TL^- to TL^+, which occurs when the lymphoid cells of TL^- mice are transformed into TL^+ leukemia cells (and is evidently due to de-repression of TL genes) is accompanied by the production of virus of any kind. Nevertheless the similarity between the two systems is enough to suggest, assuming the account of the G_{IX} system based on viral integration to be essentially true, that the Tla locus is another integrated viral genome, but in this case defective so that its only manifestation is production of antigen and leukemic

transformation. The analogy here is with defective
lysogeny in bacteria in which a phage genome becomes
defective by mutation, so that productive infection
cannot occur although other phage-specified characters
may be retained (Figure 14, and see (9)).

	circumstances associated with − ──▶ + conversion of phenotype
lysogeny: G_{IX} system	$\begin{cases} \text{production of virions} \\ \text{oncogenic transformation} \end{cases}$
defective lysogeny: TL system	oncogenic transformation

Fig. 14

* * * * * * * *

Another problem is antigenic modulation, a somewhat ominous phenomenon because it enables leukemias
to circumvent what would otherwise be a highly effective immune response. When we first observed the
anomalous appearance of TL antigen in leukemias of
TL⁻ mice, we anticipated that active immunization
against TL would protect the recipients of TL^+ leukemia
transplants, and perhaps prevent the induction of primary TL^+ leukemias, but this is not so, for the only
result of immunization is that the induced TL antibody
cancels the expression of TL antigen. From Aoki's
(unpublished) evidence, it seems the same is true of
GCSA, and there is evidence that the antigens of Burkitt's lymphoma in man are susceptible to modulation
in the same way (1,17).

It is in the TL system that most is known about
antigenic modulation, for TL modulation has been studied *in vitro*. The only other antigen that has been
similarly studied *in vitro* and has shown what seems to
be comparable modulation is the surface immunoglobulin
(Ig) which lymphocytes carry (Figure 15). Myeloma
cells, and lymphocytes of the type from which they are

ANTIGENIC MODULATION OF SURFACE Ig COMPONENTS OF
LYMPHOID CELLS

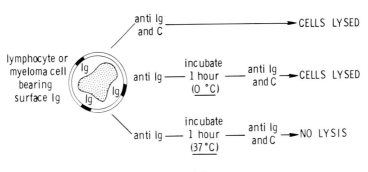

Fig. 15

derived, synthesize Ig which is incorporated in their
surfaces and can often be identified in the standard
cytotoxicity test with anti-Ig antisera. Takahashi
(21) found that pre-incubation of these cells in the
presence of anti-Ig antibody alone, with no complement
present, caused them to become completely refractory
to the later addition of complement, with or without
further anti-Ig antibody. This parallels exactly what
is seen with TL antigenic modulation *in vitro* (13).
The likely explanation of this is related to the phenomenon recently described by Raff (Figure 16 and (22)).
When lymphocytes were labeled by adding fluorescent
anti-Ig antibody in the cold the distribution of the
label was uniform over the surface of the cell. At
37°C, however, the label was gathered into patches
which then migrated to form a cap which was pincytosed,
leaving the cell bare of its immunoglobulin molecules.
Possibly the attachment of antibody to other surface
constituents like TL, GCSA or G_{IX}, has the same result,
producing antigenic modulation and defeating the homograft reaction.

There is much indication, from labeling with
immuno-ferritin, that components of the cell surface
are less fixed in position than we may have supposed,
their mobility allowing them to be specifically herded

DISAPPEARANCE OF SURFACE Ig FROM LYMPHOCYTES
EXPOSED TO ANTI-Ig ANTIBODY (Raff)

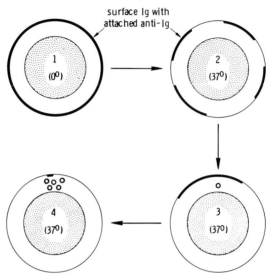

Fig. 16

together by antibody (for discussion and references
see (15)). Not all components of the cell surface are
as readily affected as TL; otherwise there would be no
histocompatibility antigens and homografts would never
be rejected.

Something resembling antigenic modulation occurs
in the ciliated unicellular organism, Paramecium. Exposure of Paramecia to antibody against a surface antigen can cause the loss of this antigen and substitu-
tion of an alternative antigen (Figure 17 and (2)).
Incidentally, serotype transformation illustrates that
Paramecia carry alternative genes, of which one is
selected for expression under a given set of conditions.
(Antibody is only one of the environmental factors that
can cause serotype transformation.) Thus the regulation of surface structure by selective gene action,
which is discussed below in relation to morphogenesis
in Metazoa, is evident even in unicellular organisms.

* * * * * * * *

SEROTYPE TRANSFORMATION IN PARAMECIUM

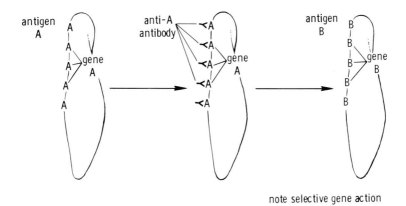

note selective gene action

Fig. 17

The next topic I will discuss has been called the "topography" of the cell surface (Review 8). Is there evidence of molecular patterning among the constituents of the cell surface? We first began to try and find out about this ourselves after observing antigenic modulation. *A priori*, we surmised that, if indeed the cell surface embodies intricate instructions for cell recognition, then there must be a high degree of order within the membrane, and if this is the case, then modulation of TL antigen by TL antibody might be accompanied by a compensatory increase in some other particular cell surface component. This, it turns out, is true; certain antigens of the H-2 locus, which is closely linked to Tla, are virtually doubled in the course of TL modulation, the representation of other antigens remaining unchanged (Figure 18). Clearly this could mean one of two things. Either the two loci are under some form of reciprocal genetic control at the chromosomal level, or else the two antigens H-2 and TL are neighbors on the cell surface, the territory occupied by TL being taken over by H-2 when TL is deleted by antibody (Figure 19). The latter would imply that there is indeed a preferential arrangement of

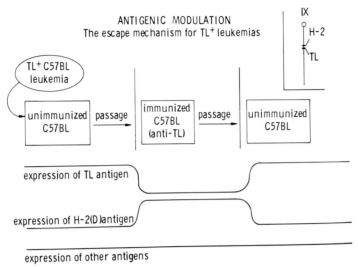

Fig. 18

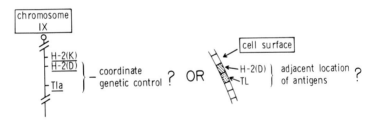

Fig. 19

different gene products on the cell surface, because
only H-2 is changed in amount as a result of modulation. H-2 and TL antigens had been isolated and chrom-
atographed by Davies, who showed that the two antigens
reside on different molecules, so it seemed safe to
conclude that we were not dealing with two different
determinants on one molecule. To find out whether
H-2 and TL are in fact neighbors on the thymocyte surface, we used the principle that if two antigens are
close enough together on the cell surface, saturation

of one of the sites with its cognate antibody impairs the uptake of antibody to the second antigen, and this can be measured in a standard quantitative absorption test.

The result was that saturation of H-2 sites with H-2 antibody produced a specific partial blocking of the uptake of TL antibody, and *vice versa*, showing that TL and H-2 antigens are indeed neighbors. This and other data made the alternative explanation of control by reciprocal gene action unlikely, and substantiated the case for an epigenetic system of positional informative to regulate the disposition of these products on the cell surface.

Use of the technique was then extended to several of the other antigens I have been discussing, in a large series of pair-by-pair comparisons. The result was that every antigen tested, and hence the molecule on which it was situated, had a definable position in relation to the others. Thus there must in fact be a map for the thymocyte surface in which each gene product has its assigned preferential position. The map shown in Figure 20 is only an illustration of the sort of arrangement that would be consistent with the blocking data. The details are not important at this stage; what is important is that there are in fact preferential patterns. Probably the positions are not fixed, which is why I use the term "preferential," because this may be inconsistent with mounting evidence that at least some components of the cell surface can migrate when bound by antibody (see discussion in (15)).

Surface patterning offers perhaps another new dimension to thoughts about morphogenesis. We have to deal with the apparent dilemma that the genome cannot contain direct instructions for the disposition of every cell in the body. Surface patterning raises the possibility that a diversity of surface arrangements might be engendered without immediate genetic specification for every cell. There is not information as to how the surface patterns we infer from our mapping studies are generated or transmitted from cell to cell, but it is worth noting that in Paramecia, regional

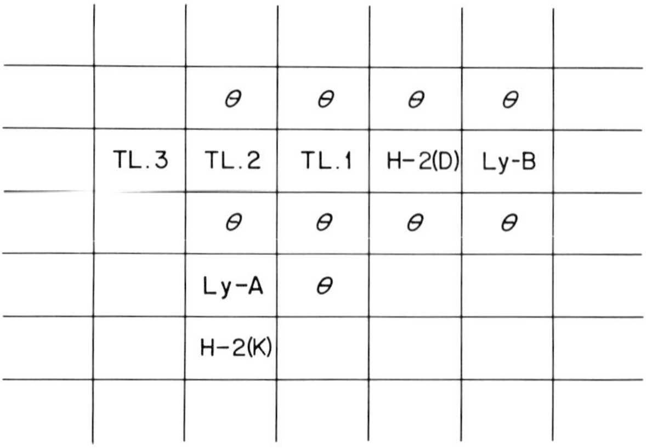

	θ	θ	θ	θ	
TL.3	TL.2	TL.1	H-2(D)	Ly-B	
	θ	θ	θ	θ	
	Ly-A	θ			
	H-2(K)				

Fig. 20: Preferential position of thymocyte surface antigens.

peculiarities of cortical structure, known as "cortical mutants," can be transmitted autonomously from generation to generation without reference to the genome (3). So, for example, one can conceive of an epigenetic mechanism for Metazoan cells which is geared to the process of cell division and results not in the copying of surface displays during each division, but in a precisely ordered series of changes in surface display. This process would generate a set of phenotypically diverse cells whose surfaces would fit together preferentially in a characteristic configuration, like a jig-saw puzzle in three dimensions. In this case the function of the genome would be reduced to selecting the correct set of genes for specifying the elements of the display on the progenitor cell of the clone.

Let me emphasize that positional information need not necessarily always, or commonly, be generated by unique inscriptions on the cell surface. There is evidence for or against this in particular contexts – I am merely commenting on a way in which such surface inscriptions *might* be generated.

What might this have to do with cancer? Conceivably a fixed tissue cell is inhibited from entering mitosis as long as its display groups over the entire surface are engaged with those of its neighbor cells. Disengagement of the surface on the death or removal of a perpetuating error in surface display may be that it becomes impossible for any progeny cell to find neighbors with which its surface can totally engage, which is the necessary condition for cessation of mitoses. How might such a display error arise in the first place? Let us consider this purely diagrammatically and imagine that the simple arrangement of of four elements, A, B, C and D shown in Figure 21 is

RECOGNITION DISPLAY USING 4 UNITS

```
A   B   C   D
B   C   D   A
C   D   A   B      Normal
D   A   B   C
```

Tolerance extends to units A, B, C and D individually But is contigent on the correct display.

Fig. 21

the correct display for a certain cell. There are at least two possibilities of error (Figure 22): first, disruption of the display by insertion of a new element, E, which we could call a genotypic error because additional genetic information is required for the specification of E; and second, alternatively, the transposition of elements in the display, which we can call a phenotypic error because, on the face of it, no new genetic information is necessary, at least not for specifying the recognition elements of the display.

Consider this now in relation to the puzzle that one class of tumor-specific transplantation antigens is so exceedingly diverse that each individual chemically-induced tumor (and the same may apply to all tumors) has a *different* one, capable of evoking a rejection response from its host. And take into account,

TWO POSSIBILITIES TO ACCOUNT FOR NEW ANTIGENICITY
OF ABERRANT DISPLAY

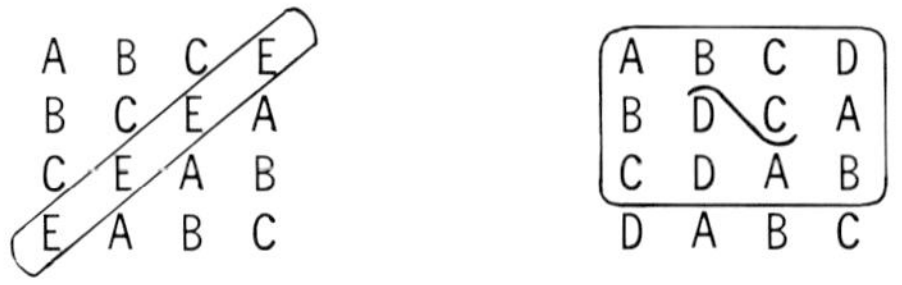

A B C E	A B C D
B C E A	B D C A
C E A B	C D A B
E A B C	D A B C

genotypic error substitutes E for D

phenotypic error transposes D and C : the new configuration generates a defect of recognition and altered antigenicity for which physiologic immunologic tolerance has made no provision.

In either case, the defect of recognition and the appearance of new antigenicity are inter-dependent.

Fig. 22

also, that these individually distinct transplantation antigens in chemically induced tumors seem in some way to be essential to malignancy. Thus, it has never been possible by immuno-selection to produce tumor lines in which they have been lost, despite the considerable disadvantage which they force upon the tumor cell, particularly in the case of highly antigenic chemically-induced tumors. In other words, malignancy seems in some way to depend on antigenicity, which is most easily explained by supposing that they are two manifestations of a single defect. Either diagram of Figure 22 is compatible with this. On the left, element E is antigenic and disrupts the recognition display. On the right, the membrane changes produced by transposition of the display elements are assumed not only to result in defective cell recognition but also to generate new antigenic groupings to which the host is not tolerant and which are therefore immunogenic.

Obviously, these particular speculations may prove to be entirely wide of the mark, but at least they emphasize that one need not assume that the appearance of new antigenicity in tumors, particularly

84

of the type that is unique for each tumor, necessarily has a genetic origin. Furthermore, they are a warning about the danger of assuming that, because malignancy is inherited by generation after generation of cancer cells, it must necessarily be due to a genetic mutation of some kind. There is no need to subscribe to that particular pre-conception. (Is it possible, for example, that preoccupation with an entirely mutational view of cancer is responsible for the fact that interest has always centered on DNA as the locus of action of chemical carcinogens, to the exclusion of the cell surface itself?) This hypothesis does not exclude that viruses play a part in the causation of some or all tumors. We are speaking now of the cellular defect immediately responsible for the malignant phenotype of the cancer cell. (For further discussion relevant to this section see (8).)

* * * * * * * *

The remarks above, about possible connections between cell surface display and morphogenesis, refer to the orientation of functionally similar cells into morphologically distinctive groups. This may be taken as the final stage of a process which began in embryogenesis with the derivation of divergent cell lineages with different functions, *i.e.*, *differentiation*, or perhaps more strictly *determination*.

I will say a little more about this in a general context, and then conclude my discussion with a few comments as to why it may be important to have these considerations in mind when studying cancer and cancer viruses. It is in the setting of cellular determination and differentiation that the θ/Ly group of differentiation antigens is particularly interesting. It is sufficiently clear that differentiation involves the selection of a particular set of genes which code for the proteins responsible for the specialized function of the cell type, such as the production of immunoglobulin by lymphocytes, hemoglobin by erythrocyte precursors, insulin by the B cells of the pancreas, and

so on.   In a word, selective gene action accounts for
specialized function.   But until recently little attention was paid to whether or not the cell surface
might likewise acquire discriminating characteristics
peculiar to particular pathways of differentiation.
With perhaps some concessions to the need for specialized surface receptors, there was a prevailing belief
that the surfaces of all cells of a particular organism
are basically very similar.   To epitomize this, if one
had asked the question of many immuno-biologists some
years ago, one would probably have received the answer
that there should be a greater correspondence of surface structure between two different cell types in one
organism than between two similar cell types in two
different organisms of the same or different species,
despite the fact that the reverse is true of the contents of the cell, *i.e.*, of the machinery of cell function.   *A priori* it is so reasonable to think that the
surface of each cell type should be coded (to a greater
or lesser extent) by special genes, to confer on each
cell type the ability to discriminate like cells from
cells following other pathways of differentiation,
that one wonders why the idea has been resisted.

Consider for example a strong argument favoring
the relation of surface constitution to cellular differentiation which comes from experiments on cell as-
sortment *in vitro* of the kind carried out particularly
by Moscona (11)(Figure 23).

In general, if two cell populations from a chick
embryo are mixed in culture with the same two cell
populations from a mouse embryo, the four cell populations first intermingle and then sort themselves out,
not according to their phylogenetic origin, chicken
vs. mouse, but according to their histogenetic type,
kidney *vs.* cartilage.   Thus, within each discrete his-
tologically-distinct grouping, cells of chicken and
mouse are intermingled.   Evidently the kidney cell
knows better that it is a kidney cell than whether it
came from a chicken or a mouse.   This is not surprising if we accept that genetic mechansims for discriminating one cell type from another were essential to

the evolution of Metazoa, and that therefore these mechanisms had been evolving already for up to a billion years before even the common ancestor of birds and mammals emerged.

RE-ASSOCIATION OF MIXED EMBRYONIC CELLS IN CULTURE:

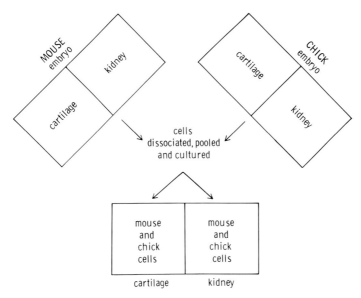

Fig. 23

The question boils down to: "Does selective gene action play a major part in specifying the surface structure of differentiated cells, as it does in specifying the function of differentiated cells, and as these cell-assortment experiments seem to imply?"

A prominent argument against it comes from transplantation biology. Hemopoietic chimeras are tolerant of tissue grafts from the donor that supplied the hemopoietic cells that colonized the recipient, as in the famous experiments of Billingham, Brent and Medawar (4), who inoculated newborn mice with foreign hemopoietic cells and later found them to be tolerant of donor skin grafts; the same is true of "radiation chimeras" produced by restoring lethally irradiated

mice with foreign bone marrow cells. This leads to
the argument that skin, for instance, does not carry
surface antigens that are lacking on hemopoietic cells,
otherwise the chimera would reject donor skin while
retaining the donor's colonizing hemopoietic cells.
The inference is that there are no special genes for
specifying surfaces of epidermal cells. One could
still say that there may be special genes for epidermal
cell surfaces, but that they are not polymorphic, *i.e.*,
not variable within the species, in which case the same
skin-specific antigen would be present on all mouse
epidermal cells and so provide no basis for rejection
of donor skin. However, as we shall see, the first
statement is partly false, so there is no immediate
need to consider the second.

Plainly we need direct proof that selective gene
action is responsible for differential surface structure. The θ and Ly systems are helpful here because
these comprise at least three genetically independent
systems whose products are expressed only or mainly
on lymphoid cells, implying that the θ and Ly genes
are repressed in all other cell types. It seems a
reasonable inference that all other cells will have
comparable differentiation antigens specified by pri-
vate sets of genes, but how can this be reconciled
with the facts of tolerance which I mentioned? Are
lymphoid cells exceptional? To make the point that
selective gene action is not a peculiarity of the specification of lymphoid cell surfaces, we choose to investigate skin because it is technically easy to work
with in the context of transplantation, and also because of the arguments that hinge on observations that
hemopoietic chimerism entails tolerance of skin grafts.
We first searched the literature for cases which might
suggest failure of skin-graft tolerance in chimeric
animals. There are in fact several such reports (cited
in (6)), and in one or two instances the authors clearly stated the possibility that rejection of donor skin
was due to skin-specific antigens, which would simply
imply selective gene action for epidermal cells. Figure 24 shows a single example. Hemopoietic chimerism

LATE REJECTION OF SKIN GRAFTS
EXCHANGED BETWEEN CHIMERIC CATTLE TWINS

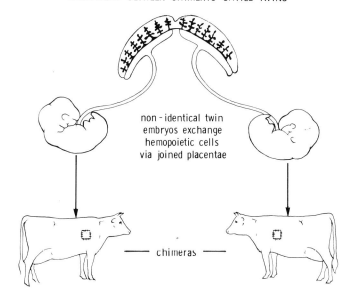

non-identical twin
embryos exchange
hemopoietic cells
via joined placentae

— chimeras —

exchanged skin grafts survive for long periods
but some are eventually rejected

Fig. 24

in cattle (14) is caused by exchange of hemopoietic
cells during fetal life *via* conjoined placentas. Such
twin chimeras possess double sets of erythrocytes and
white blood cells throughout life. They tolerate skin
grafts from one another for long periods (5), but many
of these are finally rejected (20). So acceptance of
donor skin grafts is a common but not invariable consequence of hemopoietic chimerism. Figure 25 illustrates an experimental system in mice in which detailed
study has been possible (6). Chimeras are made by
restoring lethally irradiated C57 mice with C57 x A
hemopoietic cells. In the mouse it is easy to prove
that hemopoietic chimerism exists simply by typing
erythrocytes and lymphocytes for their H-2 antigens.
Not only do such chimeras reject skin of donor type,

SKIN-SELECTIVE HOMOGRAFT REJECTION:

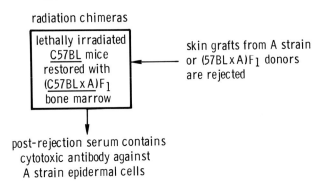

Fig. 25

but they produce antibody which is selectively cytotoxic for donor epidermal cells. So the case for selective gene action in the specialization of epidermal
cell surfaces is becoming well-substantiated. This
evidence, together with some recent serological evidence of differentiation antigens on yet other cell
types, makes a good case for selective gene action as
a general feature of cell surface differentiation. We
can even compose a rudimentary table (Figure 26) to
represent a small part of the mouse's program for differentiating the surfaces of its cell populations.
This table is from (16).

The names of all but two of the systems listed
here will I think be familar to you from what I have
said. I shall close my talk with a few comments about
cancer which are suggested by this table. The MLV-
related antigens GCSA and G_{IX} do not appear here, but
if included they would appear as primarily lymphoid
differentiation antigens like TL, θ and the Ly series;
and it is primarily in lymphoid organs that MLV makes
its appearance. Thus on the face of it the expression
of integrated leukemia virus genomes, either partially,
as in the specification of antigens independently of
virions, or completely as in productive infection,
comes under the same physiologic genetic controls that

	H-2	H-Y	Sk	θ	Pca	Ly-A	Ly-B,C	Tla
Epidermal cells	+	+	+	+	−	−	−	−
Sperm	+	+	−	−	−	−	−	−
Brain	+	+	+	+	+	−	−	−
Plasma cells	+	−	−	+	−	−	−	−
Lymphocytes	+	+	−	+	−	+	+	−
Thymocytes	+	+	−	+	−	+	+	+
Erythrocytes	+	−	−	−	−	−	−	−

+ = expressed
− = not expressed

Fig. 26: Selective gene action exemplified by the surface antigens of differentiated cells.

determine the differentiated state of the cell surface. This doubtless has to do with why a leukemia virus is a leukemia virus rather than producing some other form of cancer. So far this is clear only for leukemia, but this may be largely because we know much more about leukemogenesis than about any other form of cancer in mice. The importance of recognizing that selective gene action probably plays as large a part in differentiating the surfaces of *all* cell types as it does in the case of lymphocytes, is that we are alerted to the possibility that the expression of other oncogenic viruses and their antigens in other tissues is similarly linked to sets of genes that include among their functions the differentiation of cell surface structure. One of the main purposes of contemporary immunogenetics is to find out more about these genetic programs and how they work.

So my final comment is that in this respect, as in every other aspect I have discussed today, there may be much to be learned about the biology of cancer from systematic examination of the normal or non-malignant cell.

References

The following few citations were selected primarily for their value in providing reviews and discussions of the topics dealt with, and as keys to the literature.

1. Aoki, T., Geering, G., Beth, E., and Old, L.J. Suppression of antigen in Burkitt's lymphoma and human melanoma cells grown in selected human sera. In Recent Advances in Human Tumor Virology and Immunology, W. Nakahara, K. Nishioka, T. Harayama, and Y. Ito, eds., University of Tokyo Press, Tokyo, 1971, pp. 425–429.

2. Beale, G.H. The antigen system of *Paramecium aurelia*. In International Review of Cytology VI, G.H. Bourne and J.F. Danielli, eds., Academic Press, New York, 1957, pp. 1–23.

3. Beisson, J. and Sonneborn, T.M. Cytoplasmic inheritance of the organization of the cell cortex in *Paramecium aurelia*. Proc. Nat. Acad. Sci. 53, 275–282 (1965).

4. Billingham, R.E., Brent, L., and Medawar, P.B. 'Actively acquired tolerance' of foreign cells. Nature 172, 603–606 (1957).

5. Billingham, R.E. and Lampkin, G.H. Further studies on tissue homotransplantation in cattle. J. Embryol. Exp. Morph. 5, 351–367 (1957).

6. Boyse, E.A., Lance, E.M., Carwell, E.A., Cooper, S., and Old, L.J. Rejection of skin allografts by radiation chimaeras: selective gene action in the specification of cell surface structure. Nature 227, 901–903 (1970).

7. Boyse, E.A. and Old, L.J. Some aspects of normal and abnormal cell surface genetics. Ann. Rev. Genetics 3, 269–290 (1969).

8. Boyse, E.A. and Old, L.J. The invitation to sur-
    veillance. In Immune Surveillance, R.T. Smith
    and M. Landy, eds., Academic Press, New York,
    1970, pp. 5-30.

9. Boyse, E.A., Old, L.J., and Stockert, E. The
    relation of linkage group IX to leukemogenesis
    in the mouse. In Proceedings of the Conference
    on RNA Viruses and Host Genome in Oncogenesis.
    P. Emmelot and P. Bentvelzen, eds., North-Holland
    Publ. Co., Amsterdam, in press.

10. Gorer, P.A. and O'Gorman, P. The cytotoxic activ-
    ity of isoantibodies in mice. Transplant. Bull.
    3, 142-143 (1956).

11. Moscona, A. The development in vitro of chimeric
    aggregates of dissociated embryonic chick and
    mouse cells. Proc. Nat. Acad. Sci. 43, 184-194
    (1957).

12. Old, L.J., Boyse, E.A., and Stockert, E. The G
    (Gross) leukemia antigen. Cancer Res. 25, 813-819
    (1965).

13. Old, L.J., Stockert, E., Boyse, E.A., and Kim,
    J.H. Antigenic modulation. Loss of TL antigen
    from cells exposed to TL antibody. Study of the
    phenomenon in vitro. J. Exp. Med. 127, 523-539
    (1968).

14. Owen, R.D. Immunogentic consequences of vascular
    anastomoses between bovine twins. Science 102,
    400-401 (1945).

15. Raff, M.C. and de Petris, S. Antibody-antigen
    reactions at the lymphocyte surface: implications
    for membrane structure, lymphocyte activation and
    tolerance induction. In Proceedings, Third
    Lepetit Colloquium, London, North-Holland Publ.
    Co., Amsterdam, in press.

16. Scheid, M., Boyse, E.A., Carwell, E.A., and Old, L.J. Serologically demonstrable alloantigens of mouse epidermal cells. J. Exp. Med., in press.

17. Smith, R.T., Klein, G., Klein, E., and Clifford, P. Studies of the membrane phenomenon in cultured and biopsy cell lines from the Burkitt lymphoma. In Advances in Transplantation, J. Dausset, J. Hamburger, and G. Mathe, eds., The Williams and Wilkins Co., Baltimore, 1968, pp. 493-493; see also Smith, R.T. In Immunological Tolerance, M. Landy and W. Braun, eds., Academic Press, New York, 1969, pp. 50-52.

18. Snell, G.D. and Stimpfling, J.H. Genetics of tissue transplantation. In Biology of the Laboratory Mouse, E.L. Green, ed., McGraw Hill Book Co., New York, 2nd edition, 1966, pp. 457-491.

19. Stockert, E., Old, L.J., and Boyse, E.A. The G_{IX} system. A cell surface allo-antigen associated with murine leukemia virus; implications regarding chromosomal integration of the viral genome. J. Exp. Med. 133, 1334-1355 (1971).

20. Stone, W.H., Cragle, R.G., Swanson, E.W., and Brown, D.G. Skin grafts: delayed reaction between pairs of cattle twins showing erythrocyte chimerism. Science 148, 1335-1336 (1965).

21. Takahashi, T. Possible examples of antigenic modulation affecting H-2 antigens and cell surface immunoglobulins. Transpl. Proc. III, 1217-1220 (1971).

22. Taylor, R.B., Duffus, W.P.H., Raff, M.C., and de Petris, S. Redistribution and pinocytosis of lymphocyte surface immunoglobulin molecules induced by anti-immunoglobulin antibody. Nature New Biol. 233, 225-229 (1971).

CHEMICAL CARCINOGENESIS[*]

Emmanuel Farber[**]

Fels Research Institute
and
Departments of Pathology and Biochemistry
Temple University School of Medicine
Philadelphia, Pennsylvania 19140

It is clear today that man and animals live in a sea of carcinogens. These may be (a) agents containing translatable information, e.g. viruses, or (b) agents not containing such information but capable of altering information content of target cells, e.g. chemicals and various forms of radiation. In retrospect, it is probably significant that chemicals or mixtures of chemicals were the first causes of cancer to be recognized. This occurred some 200 years ago and since then a host of pure chemicals or mixtures have been implicated as probable or possible causes of cancer in man (Table 1) and animals. It is generally thought that well over half the cancers seen in man may be intimately related to some one or more chemicals. Even if future studies implicate viruses as playing an important or obligatory role in the development of all neoplasia, in my view this will not alter to any significant degree the importance now attached to chemicals or radiation. It will introduce a viral

---

[*] The author's research included in this survey was supported in part by research grants from the American Cancer Society (BC-7N) and the National Cancer Institute (CA 12218 and CA 10439).

[**] American Cancer Society Research Professor.

TABLE 1

SOME REPRESENTATIVE CHEMICAL AGENTS IMPLICATED
IN CANCER CAUSATION IN MAN

A. Individual Chemicals

β-Naphthylamine
Benzidine
4-amino biphenyl
Bis-chloroethyl sulfide (mustard gas)

B. Compound Classes

Asbestos
Arsenicals
Chromates

C. Radioactive Compounds

Radium
Thorotrast
Uranium ore

D. Mixtures

Tobacco and tobacco smoke
Soots
Tars

This table is from a more complete list kindly communicated to the author by Dr. Umberto Saffiotti.

step somewhere in the complex series of events between
the normal target cell and the appearance of a cancer.
Any construct, theoretical or otherwise, in which viruses become an immediate or ultimate trigger for the
neoplastic transformation must still recognize that
the chemical, at a minimum, is almost certainly needed
to set the whole sequence of carcinogenesis in motion.
In the meantime, since strong experimental evidence has
yet to be presented for an obligatory role of viruses,
we shall restrict the discussion to what chemicals may

do as the sole carcinogenic agents in the pathogenesis of cancer.

What I would like to do in this presentation is to give an overview of carcinogenesis as I see it, restricting myself almost entirely to chemical carcinogenesis and to highlight major areas of knowledge and some major gaps which must be filled. However, before doing so, it might be of interest to indicate briefly why one should be interested in carcinogenesis as a process.

There are at least four valid reasons, some practical, some conceptual, for concentrating on the study of how normal cells are altered under the influence of a carcinogen to initiate a sequence of molecular and cellular events leading to the appearance of a population of cancer cells:

(a) to prevent cancer in the face of continuing exposure to the carcinogen. Although the removal of the carcinogen from the environment is obviously the most direct and probably most effective way to conquer cancer, it may require such a rearrangement of the environment that society cannot or will not allow this to be done except slowly over decades. A knowledge of the steps in the carcinogenic process will almost certainly lead to ways to interrupt the process in the continuing presence of the carcinogen. This can be done already in a few instances in experimental animals, as we shall see later.

(b) to understand the essential nature of cancer as a basis for intelligent and rational therapy. Any population of cancer cells is already so complex as to make it highly improbable that anyone can disentangle all the threads by any approach other than an historical one.

(c) to add further tools and understanding to the biology of higher organisms. Carcinogenesis is a fascinating biological problem, the study of which will no doubt continue to add much to our knowledge about cells, their differentiation and their control.

(d) to aid in the identification of those individuals particularly susceptible to one or more forms of cancer and to prevent cancer in such individuals by removal of the carcinogenic stimulus or interrupting the process. A detailed knowledge of the steps in a carcinogenic process may very well allow such identification and possible preventive therapy.

Chemicals as initiators-- Since the isolation of pure carcinogens such as benzo(a)pyrene, from coal pitch in the 1920's (see 24), hundreds of different chemical compounds of widely different structures such as polycyclic aromatic hydrocarbons, aromatic amines, nitrosamines and nitrosamides, to name but a few groups, have been shown to be carcinogenic under one or more circumstances in may different tissues of many different species. It must be emphasized that not all the chemical carcinogens are man-made. There is an increasing list of chemicals, widely scattered in nature, that are carcinogens, sometimes even very potent ones. Included among these are aflatoxin (from some strains of *Aspergillus flavus*), pyrrolizidine alkaloids (in many plants-senicio, crotolaria, etc.), cycasin (in primitive palm trees, e.g. *cycad circinalis*) and safrole (in oil of sassafras). In an early attempt to arrive at some valid generalization concerning the underlying basis for the common biological response to such a diversity of chemical structures, Haddow suggested many years ago that many chemicals were alkylating agents or converted to alkylating agents by the body. Work during the past 15 years or so by a number of laboratories around the world, spearheaded by the outstanding work of the Millers (21) has given solid verification for this suggestion and has placed the initial step in chemical carcinogenesis on a firm foundation of fact. As "synthesized" by the Millers (21,22), the majority if not all chemical carcinogens are either electrophilic reactants *per se* or converted to such active derivatives, called ultimate carcinogens, by enzymes in the appropriate target tissues. In the case of at least some direct acting compounds such as nitrosamides, their reactivity as electrophilic reactants is greatly enhanced by cysteine, glutathione or possibly other SH containing compounds in the target cells. Some representative carcinogens

and their active metabolic derivatives are shown in
Figs. 1 and 2. Those in Fig. 1 are the electrophilic
reactants *per se* and seem to be active without any
prior metabolism. The "procarcinogens" in Fig. 2 are
the compounds usually present in the environment and
require metabolic conversion to an active electrophilic
reactant before they are carcinogenic.

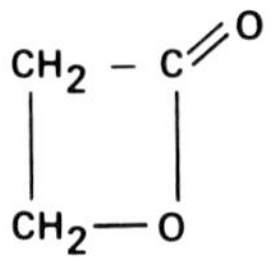

β – PROPIOLACTONE

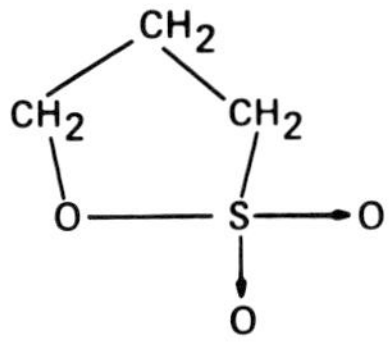

PROPANESULTONE

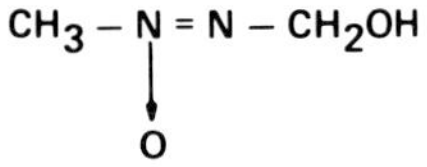

$CH_3 - N = N - CH_2OH$

METHYLAZOXYMETHANOL

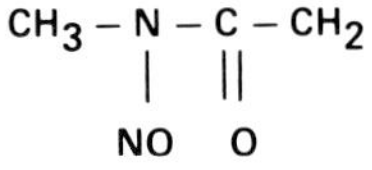

$CH_3 - N - C - CH_2$

N – METHYL – N – NITROSOUREA

$CH_3 - N - C - N - NO_2$

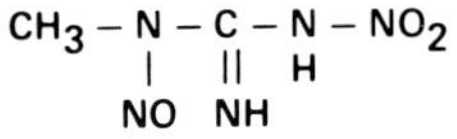

N – METHY – N^1 – NITRO – N – NITROSOGUANIDINE

Fig. 1: Some representative examples of carcinogens
in which the carcinogen as used is the electrophilic
reactant.

In most instances, the enzymes involved are microsomal and at least some are in the mixed function oxi-
dase group. As with other microsomal enzymes, little
progress has been made in the isolation, purification
and characterization of these enzymes. A new enzymatic
activity, N-hydroxylation, was discovered during the
study of the metabolism of 2-acetylaminofluorene (2-AAF)
and this lead in turn to the more recent work on the
nature of the ultimate carcinogens (21). Because of
their high chemical reactivity, the compounds closest

chemically to the ultimate carcinogen become increasingly difficult to work with. One interesting development is the probable role of enzymes such as sulfotransferase which catalyzes the reaction of N-hydroxy-2-AAF with 3'-phosphoadenosyl-5'phosphosulfate (PAPS) to form the sulfate ester of N-hydroxy-2-AAF, a very potent electrophilic reactant (21,22).

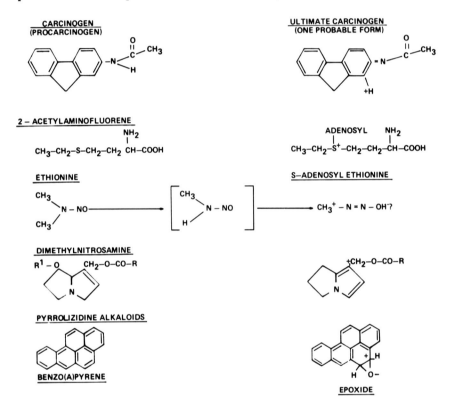

Fig. 2: Some examples of carcinogens ("procarcinogens") which require metabolic conversion to an active form (ultimate carcinogen).

The levels of activities can be modulated by a variety of drugs, dietary modifications, etc. It must be remembered that the concept of drug-induced enzymes and the possible importance of such induction in the analysis of the biological effects of drugs and toxic compounds was suggested from the early studies on chemical carcinogenesis (6,22).

In addition to producing a more active derivative, many enzymes, again mainly microsomal, produce a less active or inactive derivative. This is especially true with the aromatic amines and other aromatic or heterocyclic carcinogens but may not be true for aliphatic compounds such as many of the nitrosamines. Quantitatively, the degree of inactivation is far greater than that of activation, the latter amounting to no more than a few percent at most (see 22,30). The balance between the activities of the inactivating and the activating enzymes thus becomes one of the first critical steps in carcinogenesis with many carcinogens. By inducing an increase in the levels of inactivation by drugs, such as with phenobarbital or 3-methylcholanthrene in the case of the liver and benzoflavones and others in the case of skin, etc., one can effectively block cancer induction, often completely, with several carcinogens (e.g. see 11,22,25,26). This clear-cut experimental demonstration of the prevention of cancer in the continuing presence of the carcinogen becomes a potentially exciting model for the ultimate application to man in selected situations, e.g. groups at high risk for some types of cancer because of occupation, habit patterns (e.g. smoking) or some underlying disease.

It must be emphasized that the tissue distribution of the different enzymes acting on carcinogens is quite varied, some cells or organs being very active and others less so or even inactive. This is also true in different species. These distribution patterns are no doubt responsible for some of the organ and species specificity seen with many carcinogens. The clarification of the enzymology and tissue distribution for the different enzymes should allow increasingly accurate prediction of what tissues may or may not be target organs for specific carcinogens in different species but especially in man.

An interesting recent development concerns the
de novo generation in the body of nitrosamines from
dietary amines and nitrite (e.g. 23). It has been
clearly shown that a variety of nitrosamines active as
carcinogens can be synthesized in the gastrointestinal
tract of experimental animals from secondary amines and
nitrite added to the diet. Although the levels used
experimentally were of necessity higher than those that
would be found naturally, nevertheless the principle is
very important. This is especially true with nitrosamines which are generally easily synthesized and are
such versatile carcinogens for so many different tissues and species (19). Increasing concern has been
expressed about the possible importance in cancer induction of the nitrites added so often to foods, especially meat and meat products (16).

Effects of activated carcinogens on host targets--
Given a chemically reactive form of a carcinogen in
certain types of cells, it is not at all surprising
that this will react with many different nucleophiles
present in cells. Thus, virtually all chemical carcinogens react covalently with DNA, RNA and protein
and probably with other macromolecules such as some
polysaccharides under some circumstances (see 9,10).
In DNA and RNA, the major site of reaction with many
carcinogens (e.g. nitrosamines, nitrosamides, β-pro-
priolactone, aromatic amines) is N-7 or C-8 of guanine.
However, under a variety of circumstances, many other
sites of reaction have been described (12). These include N-3 and 0-6 of guanine, N-1, N-3 and N-7 of
adenine and N-1 of cytosine (12). For example, with
all methylating and ethylating agents studied, the
major product of their reaction with DNA and RNA is
7-methylguanine (Fig. 3). This usually amounts to
from 70 to 90% of the methylation of DNA (12). However, smaller and more variable degrees of alkylation
of all the other available N atoms in purines have been
reported several times. With aromatic amines, especially 2-AAF, the major site of reaction is C-8 of
guanine (Fig. 4).

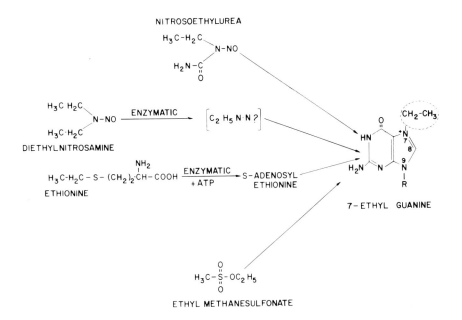

Fig. 3: The production of 7–ethylguanine as a type reaction between two direct ethylating agents (nitrosoethylurea, ethylethanesulfonate) and two indirect ethylating carcinogens (diethylnitrosamine, ethionine) and DNA or RNA.

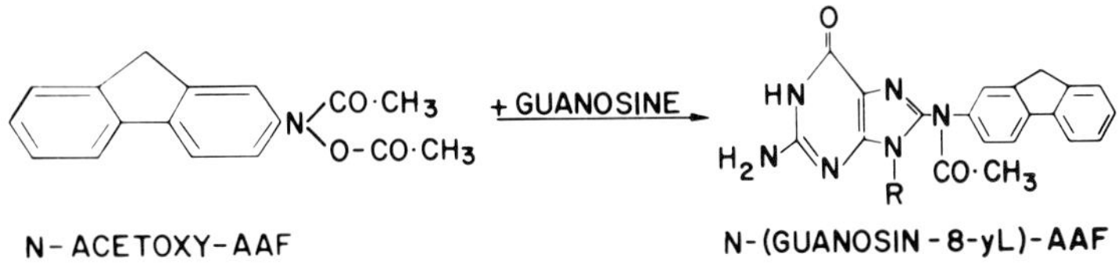

Fig. 4: The reaction between an active form of the carcinogen, 2-AAF (N–acetoxy-AAF) and guanosine to form N-(guanosin-8-yl)-AAF.

The patterns of reaction with different RNA's vary with the carcinogen. Some, e.g. ethionine and to a lesser degree 2-acetylaminofluorene (2-AAF) react mostly with tRNA (29). Others, e.g. dimethylnitrosamine, seem to be less selective. So far, no studies indicating selective or non-selective interaction with different fractions of DNA (more or less redundant, more or less active as template for RNA synthesis, etc.) have been reported. In protein, several amino acids, such as histidine (19), methionine, cysteine, tryptophane and tyrosine (21) appear to be especially reactive with different carcinogens.

These effects on macromolecules naturally are reflected in alterations at higher levels of organization - membranes of the endoplasmic reticulum, mitochondria, nucleoli, etc. (see 10).

Thus, not unexpectedly, the generation of chemically highly reactive moieties from chemical carcinogens leads to many reactions in those cells susceptible to or generating the active components (Fig. 5). This plethora of chemical effects naturally makes the choice of biological relevance difficult. However, the availability of a variety of different chemicals active as

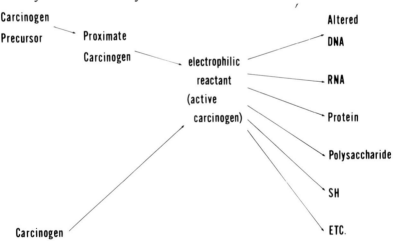

Fig. 5: Schematic representation of initial interactions between chemical carcinogens and target cells. The carcinogen precursor is the compound as usually administered which must be converted to an active form, the proximate or ultimate carcinogens, to be active in initiation of carcinogenesis.

carcinogens, the increasing body of information concerning the details of the specific reactions involved and their similarities and differences and the many common features seen in the subsequent cellular responses during carcinogenesis offer many opportunities to probe in increasing depth into the next major question - which reactions and effects are pertinent and mechanistically important to the further steps in the induction of cancer and which are irrelevant. I shall return to this important aspect later.

The Cancer Cell - biological and biochemical properties-- Before discussing the next steps in the carcinogenic process, I would like to jump to the end of the line - the cancer cell - in the hope that a brief discourse about the properties of the end result of a carcinogenic process may help us to obtain a better perspective of the whole progression.

The hallmarks of a cancer that allow us to identify it as such are the ability of the cells to *grow, invade* and *metastasize* (Table 2). These behavioral patterns are almost always accompanied by cytologic aberrations, especially of the cell nucleus. Biologically, these are not a tightly coupled package but are almost certainly *separate units of aberration*. Thus, many early precancerous lesions may show cytologic aberrations with some growth without invasion or metastasis. Also cancers of different tissues or at different times in their life history may show growth, growth with invasion or growth with invasion with metastasis. Again, some neoplasms, such as basal cell carcinoma, may show extensive growth and invasion, even to the point of killing the patient, without any evidence for metastasis. Of course part of these differences may reside in variations in the host response, e.g. immunologic. However, it is well documented that populations of cells may show some of the changes without the others as inherent properties in the cells themselves. It must be realized in this context that usually there is some apparent sequence - growth, then invasion and then metastasis. Also, growth is not a single element - it may be very slow or very rapid or any level between these extremes.

TABLE 2

THE CANCER CELL - SOME CHARACTERISTIC PROPERTIES

A. Biological

Growth
Invasion
Metastasis
Cytologic aberration, *e.g.* nuclear

B. Biochemical

Apparently inappropriate expression of
genetic information

(1) Hormones, *e.g.* ACTH, parathormone
(2) Isozymes, *e.g.* hexokinase, aldolase,
pyruvate kinase, adenylate kinase
(3) Fetal proteins, *e.g.* gastrointestinal,
carcinoembryonic antigen, liver alpha
fetoprotein

Obviously, these properties will not be understood
until we clarify their underlying mechanisms. However,
from the vantage point of today, it appears most likely
that in cancer, we have a package of separate units of
change, each with its characteristic underlying biochemical basis. If this is valid, then we cannot hope
to learn too much about the metabolic and molecular
mechanisms responsible for each of the behavior patterns by studying them as part of a complex package in
a fully formed cancer.

As yet, it is virtually impossible to relate the
well known surface changes of neoplastic cells *in vitro*
to any of the biological properties discussed here.
So-called contact inhibition itself remains a puzzling
phenomenon whose very existence has been placed in doubt
by recent work of Holley and others on serum growth
factors. Hopefully, the clarification of this phenomenon at some mechanistic level and the exciting newer
developments on membrane biology and biochemistry in

normal and neoplastic cells may allow some extrapolation to invasion and metastasis as manifestations of cancer cells growing in a live host. The study of the control of growth of cells is now being actively pursued in many laboratories. The cell cycle and its sequence of steps, the correlation between differences in chromatin activity in transcription and the probable importance of non-histone proteins in different stages of the cell cycle offer the prospect of some real understanding of the growth component of a cancer (see 2).

However, despite these advances, the nub of the problem as it relates to cancer is still unclear – *what controls growth in vivo* and *how is it modulated quantitatively? What properties control the spread of cells, both locally and distantly?*

In looking at the progress in the study of the biochemistry of cancer, we are faced on the one hand with a bewildering array of isolated facts that add up at best to the conclusion that neoplastic behavior is compatible with many different metabolic patterns at the phenotypic level and on the other hand with some emerging generalizations – namely, that cancer cells as a group show what appears to be *inappropriate expression of genetic information.* This is manifest in many different human and chemically induced experimental cancers in at least three ways (Table 2).

(a) <u>Hormone</u> <u>production</u> – many neoplasms produce and secrete hormones, e.g. ACTH, parathormone, and possibly insulin and erythropoetin even though the tissue of origin does not (e.g. 5,17).

(b) <u>Isozymes</u> – many neoplasms show activities of isozymes of several enzymes not seen in the tissue of origin (e.g. 7,27,28), and

(c) <u>Fetal</u> <u>proteins</u> – an increasing number of cancers produce proteins, such as gastrointestinal carcinoembryonic antigens and liver alpha-fetoglobulins, which were characteristic at the fetal stage of development (e.g. 1).

Although none of these are constant accompaniments of neoplasia of any single organ or cell, they are nevertheless so common as to indicate a fundamental alteration in gene expression in cancer. At present, this manifestation seems *inappropriate* for the state of differentiation of the neoplastic cells. However, this conclusion could be merely a concomitant of our basic ignorance in relating biochemical and metabolic activity to biological behavior in cells in general. Parenthetically, it should be pointed out that these new expressions of patterns of protein synthesis are proving to be increasingly useful as diagnostic aids in human cancer.

The carcinogenic process-- Given (a) a *highly reactive chemical* able to effect one or more of the many different chemical changes in DNA, (b) the *mutagenic action* of several ultimate carcinogens in bacteria and bacteriophage (20), and (c) the *altered gene expression* as a fundamental characteristic of neoplastic cells, it follows that an attractive hypothesis for carcinogenesis is as follows (Fig. 6): the ultimate

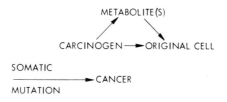

Fig. 6: Schematic representation of carcinogenesis, hypothesis I.

carcinogen acting on a population of target cells converts a small population to a neoplastic state via a process analogous to a somatic mutation. Everything else merely modulates the expression of this fundamentally simple process. Since the number of genes involved in the control of cell behavior, especially as

it relates to growth, may be large, one could imagine
that a large number of the phenotypic variations seen
in cancer are epiphenomena, not intimately involved
in the changes essential for neoplasia. This simplis-
tic view of neoplasia is especially appealing to those
of us who like to think chemically, i.e. in terms of
their identifiable chemical events, hopefully few in
type, that are the underlying basis for the development of cancer.

However, the *facts do not support this straight-
forward* one-step process. In 1940, Rous and Berenblum
and their coworkers (see 3,4) showed clearly that the
carcinogenic process is divisible into *at least two*
steps – called *initiation* and *promotion* or *co-carcino-
genesis*.

However, this can be reconciled with hypothesis I
by inserting another step – the dormant cancer cell
that has to be awakened by promoter or co-carcinogen
(hypothesis II - Fig. 7). One can even introduce a

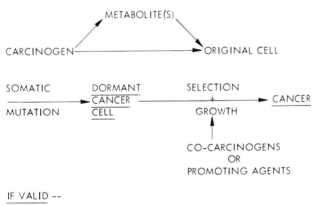

Fig. 7: Schematic representation of carcinogenesis,
hypothesis II.

more sophisticated component into the sequence - selection, for which there appears to be ample suspicion

and which ties in well with current thoughts on immunologic surveillance in carcinogenesis. The formulation of carcinogenesis in terms of the sequence-initiation-(dormancy, selection)-promotion is a favorite hypothesis today among workers in carcinogenesis.

However, here again, the facts are not compatible with this thesis. According to this view, the limiting or rate-limiting step in carcinogenesis in many tissues is cell proliferation. If this can be induced, somehow, we have in hypothesis II all the key *positive* ingredients for carcinogenesis providing the *negative* ones such as repair and immunologic surveillance are suppressed or bypassed. This hypothesis suggests that given (a) the interactions between the carcinogen and the target cell and (b) a stimulus for cell proliferation, the first cell to grow out would be the dormant cancer cell. However, in many carcinogenic processes, the first cell to grow out is not a cancer cell but a relatively normal appearing and normal behaving cell which grows and may continue to do so for a relatively long period of time, weeks or months, as compared to the initiation process which may last only hours or a few days. Cancer appears only much later in the time sequence - anywhere from two to six months or longer. Also, one can induce by appropriate means intense proliferation in skin following initiation by the application of a carcinogen without any effect on cancer induction.

Since this non-neoplastic proliferative response is such a striking component in carcinogenesis, I think it deserves a little more attention. In many carcinogenic processes, both human and animal, one sees localized cell proliferation as a striking feature before and sometimes long before one sees cancer. This is seen in skin, mammary gland, liver and some other systems (Figs. 8,9). Let me illustrate this by discussing briefly the development of hyperplastic nodules in liver (10). With virually every carcinogen, one sees innumerable such localized areas of cell proliferation many weeks before any evidence of cancer appears. There is evidence that each nodule may be a clone that is being selected for growth.

110

A. CARCINOMA-IN-SITU - HUMAN AND ANIMAL

SKIN
CERVIX
UTERINE BODY
BREAST
ETC.

CYTOLOGIC CHANGES AND GROWTH BUT NO INVASION OR METASTASIS

B. BENIGN NEOPLASMS ⟶ CANCER (HUMAN)

GROWTH WITHOUT CYTOLOGIC ABERRATION, INVASION OR METASTASIS

C. ANIMAL MODELS

ORIGINAL TISSUE CELLS ⟶ GROWTH ⟶ CANCER

Fig. 8: Some examples from human and animal experience of proliferative lesions as probable precursors
for cancer.

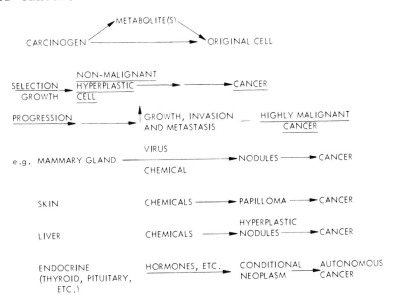

Fig. 9: Schematic representation of carcinogenesis,
hypothesis III.

This new non-cancerous cell population arising as
scattered foci throughout the liver, is seen regularly
under a wide variety of conditions associated with

111

carcinogenesis. Of course, these may all be phenomena parallel to the development of cancer and not directly related to cancer as precursors. In the liver, however, we do have evidence for these new populations being precursors (10):

(a) With a wide *variety of hepatotoxic agents*, only agents which induce *hyperplastic nodules induce liver cancer*. However, this could still be two parallel paths and not a single linear one.

(b) If the dietary conditions are so manipulated as to favor very large nodules, one can see cancer arising in nodules without a detectable cancer in any non-hyperplastic tissue.

(c) The hyperplastic nodules induced with one carcinogen, 2-acetylaminofluorene (2-AAF), show the persistence of bound carcinogen in glycogen even when the AAF has been removed from the diet weeks before. No bound carcinogen was found in the glycogen of the surrounding non-nodular liver. With AAF, the small amount of glycogen in the liver cancers also shows bound AAF even though none is found in the surrounding liver and even though the animals have not been exposed to the AAF for 4 months or longer. Thus, there are 3 lines of evidence to suggest that the hyperplastic nodule in liver, at least with one potent carcinogen, AAF, is a precursor lesion for cancer.

Given these considerations, we must now entertain a revised hypothesis (hypothesis III) for carcinogenesis (Fig. 9). Here we have introduced further steps between initiation and the cancer cell. However, we have done more - we have interrupted the cellular continuity. We now introduce a discontinuity by adding at least one or probably several new cell populations which do not have the properties seen in an obvious cancer and do not behave like "respectable" cancer cells.

There is evidence that these nodules are both homogeneous in some parameters and heterogeneous in others (10). Some nodules are readily reversible when the carcinogen is removed and others are much less so or perhaps are even irreversible. Also, we have found common patterns of disturbed glycogen and carbohydrate metabolism in virtually all nodules induced by 3 different carcinogens - ethionine, aflatoxin B_1 and 2-AAF. Becker and his colleagues have found evidence for heterogenicity - different nodules have different patterns of production of different serum proteins (see 10). All of these differences and similarities could be due to differences in the environment and not really inherent properties of the new cell populations. This is a difficult but very important phase of carcinogenesis since the answer found could clearly point to one or another mechanism operating.

Further study of this new population of cells that seem to be obligatory precursors of liver cancer indicates the existence of at least two different kinds. The first, called population II (see Fig. 10), is reversible and is dependent upon the continued exposure to carcinogen for growth. Following removal of the carcinogen from the environment, this population ceases to grow and regresses, apparently completely. The second, population III (Fig. 10), seems to evolve from population II, is no longer carcinogen-dependent and has acquired a moderate degree of autonomy in regard to growth and survival.

Thus, our current hypothesis of carcinogenesis, restricted so far to the liver, is portrayed schematically in Fig. 10. Central to this proposal is the thesis that during carcinogenesis we are dealing with a series of selections of new populations for properties that have survival value in the organism. For example, there is now increasing evidence (see 10) beginning with the work of Laws and of Stich and Maini about 15 years ago, that carcinogens, including hepatic carcinogens, have a striking inhibitory effect on both mitosis and DNA synthesis. If one stimulates liver cell proliferation by partial hepatectomy, the carcinogen-fed rat responds poorly or not at all by regeneration on the part of the original liver cells. However, the cells of the hyperplastic nodule are very responsive. Thus, the treatment with carcinogen has now selected out a more resistant population that no longer

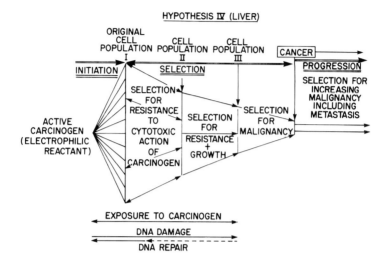

Fig. 10: Current working hypothesis of liver carcinogenesis, based on two key types of reactions – an initial alteration in pivotal target cell macromolecules
by an activated form of a carcinogen and the subsequent
progressive selection of cell populations for resistance
to cytotoxicity, autonomous growth and malignancy.

shows the carcinogen-induced inhibitory phenomenon seen
in the original cell population. In line with this,
we have obtained increasing evidence that the hyperplastic cell population is resitant to the acute cytotoxic effect of a carcinogen such as dimethylnitrosamine (DMN) even though the hyperplastic cells take up
DMN to a degree equal to that of normal liver cells
and methylate DNA and RNA to the same extent. In addition, there is evidence for some interference with the
uptake by the nodule cells of a lipid soluble carcinogen such as 2-AAF. Virtually every nodule in the liver,
induced by any one of a dozen or more different chemical carcinogens, shows a characteristic biochemical
lesion – resistance of part of the glycogen to breakdown on fasting and to glucagon administration. This
is associated with low glycogen phosphorylase and glu-
cose-6-phosphatase activity levels in the nodules. All

of these findings raise the interesting possibility
that the hyperplastic cell population may have developed some defect in the metabolism of cyclic AMP. The
failure to respond to glucagon, the altered uptake of
a lipid soluble carcinogen, 2-AAF, and the altered
glycogen phosphorylase levels seem to suggest that the
new cell populations, II and III, may have some dis-
turbance in one of its communication systems with the
environment. Whether this involves alteration in their
cell surface properties including that portion relating
to cyclic AMP and appropriate receptors, changes in the
binding proteins for some carcinogens (see 18) or in
the further metabolic use of cyclic AMP remain interesting and now experimentally approachable areas for
intensive study.

Thus, what is emerging from all of these studies
is a more realistic conception of carcinogenesis as a
process of *cellular* or *micro-evolution*. According to
this concept, a carcinogen has at least two important
properties – to change the information content of a
target cell by covalent interaction with those cellular macromolecules involved in determining the potential metabolic behavior, e.g. DNA, etc. and to create
an environment which exerts selection pressure for
certain types of cells and not for others. In an organ
such as the liver which consists predominantly of resting cells, at least two populations of cells may have
to be selected for – firstly, a population which is
resistant to the cytotoxic effects of the environment
and secondly, a population not only resistant to the
inhibitory influence of the environment but now also
possessing the property of more or less autonomous
growth (Fig. 10). The continual growth of such cells,
previously damaged by the effects of the active carcinogen on key macromolecules, such as DNA, has set
the stage for the further evolution by selection to a
population with neoplastic properties. In the case of
at least one carcinogen, 2-AAF, persistence in the new
cell populations of the original damage to DNA can be
seen with the electron microscope, which shows obvious
distortion of the orderly double-strand structures seen
in normal liver cells (Fig. 11).

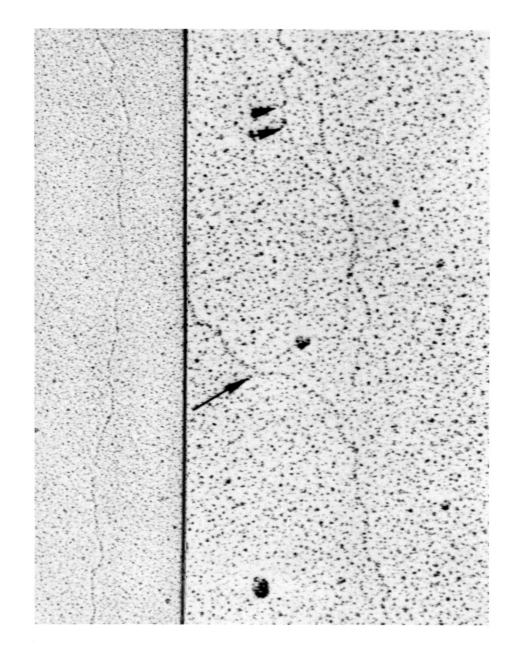

Fig. 11: Electron microscopic view of DNA isolated from normal rat liver (above) and from hyperplastic liver nodules induced by 2-AAF (below). Note the long linear double-strand molecule from the normal animal and the strand separation with unusual arrangement of single strands in the nodule DNA. Other portions of the nodule DNA showed areas of irregular "puddles" and twisted masses, mostly single-stranded (8).

In other organs in which part of the original cell population shows continual but controlled growth, the steps leading to the selection of a population autonomous for growth may well be different and may require fewer stages. However, the available evidence is consistent with the essential usefulness of this type of dynamic evolutionary approach to carcinogenesis.

Obviously, no clear-cut definition of the nature of the molecular lesions essential for any neoplastic transformation is possible until we understand much more about the molecular basis for cell differentiation and cell growth. How can cells within the same organism, e.g. neurones, hepatocytes, myocardial cells, etc. show such striking differences in organization and function and yet presumably have the same information content? The clarification of this puzzling phenomenon is fundamental to any understanding of cancer. However, there is room for many fundamental studies of cellular biochemistry in carcinogenesis until we are able to come to grips with this key essential problem in cell biology.

One such study concerns repair mechanisms of cell damaged by carcinogens. The cell is by no means a passive target for active forms of carcinogens but on the contrary has many metabolic patterns with which it can overcome at least some of the damaging effects of the cancer-inducing agents. One such concerns the damage to DNA. As discussed previously by Dr. Cleaver in this volume, DNA repair is believed to be an important phenomenom in the genesis of skin cancer and in the unusual susceptibility to cancer development of

patients with xeroderma pigmentosum. As indicated
above, there is evidence that altered DNA may be present in the new cell populations that appear to be precursors for cancer in the liver. These considerations
have prompted us to undertake systematic studies of
the patterns and mechanisms of DNA damage and repair
under the influence of chemical carcinogens. Initially,
my colleague, Dr. Lieberman, began these studies with
a human cell population, lymphocytes, and these have
already given us some insight into the interaction between various chemical carcinogens and DNA (13-15).
More recently, my colleague, Dr. Sarma, has developed
a way to study this in liver. This has the advantage
that we can now, for the first time, focus our attention on cells that, unlike lymphocytes, are the tar-
gets for cancer development by a variety of chemical
carcinogens. With this newer system, we can now begin to ask many questions that may have a direct relevance to carcinogenesis. Although this work is still
in its early stages, it is already evident that carcinogens induce extensive damage to liver DNA and that
the patterns of repair of such damage vary with the
nature of the carcinogen. An attractive hypothesis
for which we now have some evidence relates the induction of double-strand damage by a chemical to its carcinogenicity. This approach may enable us to begin
to understand why procedures such as partial hepatectomy may have an important effect in enabling liver
cancer induction with a single dose of a carcinogen.

Regardless of whether or not DNA proves to be the
sole or major molecular target for chemical carcinogens, it is already evident that we shall learn much
about this dynamic repository of information in cells
of higher organisms through this approach.

As emphasized above, we do not think that one
can realistically study carcinogenesis by concentrating entirely upon the initial molecular alterations in
target cells, since the fate of the cells containing
such alterations is very much a function of the host
and organ environment. Included in environmental factors are not only the local ones but also systematic
ones, such as immunologic. The continual removal of

altered cells that may be potential precursors for cancer by immunologic systems, called immunologic surveillance, is probably a key environmental factor in the resistance of an organism to neoplastic development. Although the existence of such a surveillance mechanism is highly probable, its exact role in any phase of carcinogenesis, especially the early ones, has yet to be delineated in any precise way. Hopefully, with clearer definition of the various cell populations during cancer induction, it may become possible to devise more critical ways to determine the exact role of immunologic surveillance in carcinogenesis.

Finally, reference must be made to the newer developments in chemical carcinogenesis *in vitro*. Many of the questions that will require clarification for any understanding of chemical carcinogenesis will no doubt come from studies *in vitro*. The work of Sachs, DiPaolo and Heidelberger and their coworkers has begun to lay solid experimental foundation for this approach to carcinogenesis. Unfortunately, we still lack systems in which questions posed by observations *in vivo* may be posed in an *in vitro* system composed of a similar cell population and vice versa. Hopefully, as the *in vitro* field is expanded and especially as epithelial cells, such as from liver, will be used, we should begin to create essential bridges between *in vitro* and comparable *in vivo* systems for carcinogenesis.

Acknowledgements

The author wishes to express his sincere thanks to Mrs. Barbara Dole for her assistance in the preparation of this manuscript.

References

1. Abelev, G.I. Alpha-Fetoprotein in ontogenesis and its association with malignant tumors. Adv. Cancer Res. 14, 295 (1971).

2. Baserga, R. The Cell Cycle and Cancer, Marcel Dekker, Inc., New York, 1971.

3. Berenblum, I. The two-stage mechanism of carcinogenesis as an analytical tool, in Cellular Control Mechanisms and Cancer, O. Mühlbock and P. Emmelot (eds.), Elsevier Publishing Co., Amsterdam, 1964.

4. Boutwell, R.K. Some biological aspects of skin carcinogenesis. Prog. Exptl. Tumor Res. 4, 207 (1964).

5. Bower, B.F. and Gordan, G.S. Hormonal effects of non-endocrine tumors. Ann. Rev. Med. 16, 83 (1965).

6. Conney, A.H., Miller, E.C. and Miller, J.A. The metabolism of methylated azo dyes. V. Evidence for induction of enzyme synthesis in the rat by 3-methylcholanthrene. Cancer Res. 16, 450 (1956).

7. Cris, W.E. A review of isozymes in cancer. Cancer Res. 31, 1523 (1971).

8. Epstein, S.M., Benedetti, E.L., Shinozuka, H., Bartus, B. and Farber, E. Altered and distorted DNA from a premalignant liver lesion induced by 2-fluorenylacetamide. Chem.-Biol. Interactions 1, 113 (1969-70).

9. Farber, E. Studies on the molecular mechanisms of carcinogenesis, in Homologies in Enzymes and Metabolic Pathways: Metabolic Alterations in Cancer, W.H. Whelan and J. Schultz (eds.), North-Holland Publishing Co., Amsterdam, 1970.

10. Farber, E. Hyperplastic liver nodules. Methods in Cancer Research 7, 1972, in press.

11. Gelboin, H.V., Wiebel, F. and Diamond, L. Dimethylbenzanthracene tumorgenesis and aryl hydrocarbon in mouse skin: inhibition by 7,8 benzoflavone. Science 170, 169 (1970).

12. Lawley, P.D. Effects of some chemical mutagens and carcinogens on nucleic acids. Prog. Nucleic Acid Res. Mol. Biol. 5, 89 (1966).

13. Lieberman, M.W., Baney, R.N., Lee, R.E., Sell, S. and Farber, E. Studies on DNA repair in human lymphocytes treated with proximate carcinogens and alkylating agents. Cancer Res. 31, 1297 (1971).

14. Lieberman, M.W., Sell, S. and Farber, E. Deoxyribonucleoside incorporation and the role of hydroxyurea in a model lymphocyte system for studying DNA repair in carcinogenesis. Cancer Res. 31, 1307 (1971).

15. Lieberman, M.W., Rutman, J.Z. and Farber, E. Thymidine labeling of pyrimidine isostichs from human lymphocyte DNA during repair after damage with N-acetoxy acetylaminofluorene or nitrogen mustard. Biochim. Biophys. Acta 247, 497 (1971).

16. Lijinsky, W. and Epstein, S.S. Nitrosamines as environmental carcinogens. Nature 225, 21 (1970).

17. Lipsett, M.B. Hormonal syndromes associated with neoplasia. Adv. Metabol. Disorders 3, 111 (1968).

18. Litwack, G., Morey, K.S. and Ketterer, B., Corticosteroid binding proteins of liver cytosol and interactions with carcinogens, in Effect of Drugs on Cellular Control Mechanisms, B.R. Rabin and R.B. Freedman (eds.), Macmillan, London, 1972.

19. Magee, P.N. and Barnes, J.M. Carcinogenic nitroso compounds. Adv. Cancer Res. 10, 163 (1967).

20. Miller, E.C. and Miller, J.A. The mutagenicity of chemical carcinogens: correlations, problems and interpretations, in Chemical Mutagens, A. Hollander (ed.), Vol. 1, Plenum Press, New York, London, 1971.

21. Miller, J.A. Carcinogenesis by chemicals: an overview - G.H.A. Clowes Memorial Lecture. Cancer Res. 30, 559 (1970).

22. Miller, J.A. and Miller, E.C. Chemical carcinogenesis: mechanisms and approaches to its control. J. Natl. Cancer Inst. 47, V (1971).

23. Sander, J. and Burkle, G. Induktion maligner Tumoren bei Ratten durch gleichzeitige Verfütterung von Vitrit und sekundären Aminen. Z. Krebsforsch. 73, 54 (1969).

24. Shimkin, M.B. and Triolo, V.A. History of carcinogenesis: some prospective remarks, in Carcinogenesis: A Broad Critique, Twentieth Annual Symposium on Fundamental Cancer Research at the University of Texas and M.D. Anderson Hospital and Tumor Institute, Williams and Wilkins, Baltimore, 1967.

25. Wattenberg, L.W. Chemoprophylaxis of carcinogenesis: a review. Cancer Res. 26, 1520 (1966).

26. Wattenberg, L.W. Enzymatic reactions and carcinogenesis, in Environment and Cancer, Twenty-fourth Annual Symposium on Fundamental Research at the University of Texas and M.D. Anderson Hospital and Tumor Institute, Williams and Wilkins, Baltimore, 1971.

27. Weinhouse, S. Respiration, glycolysis and enzyme alterations in liver neoplasms, in Homologies in Enzyme and Metabolic Pathways: Metabolic Alterations in Cancer, W.H. Whelan and J. Schultz (eds.), North-Holland Publishing Co., Amsterdam, 1970.

28. Weinhouse, S. Glycolysis, respiration and anomalous gene expression in experimental hepatomas - G.H.A. Clowes Memorial Lecture. Cancer Res. 32, 2007 (1972).

29. Weinstein, I.B. Modifications in transfer RNA during chemical carcinogenesis, in Genetic Concepts and Neoplasia, Twenty-third Annual Symposium on Fundamental Cancer Research at the University of Texas and M.D. Anderson Hospital and Tumor Institute, Williams and Wilkins, Baltimore, 1970.

30. Weisburger, E.K. and Weisburger, J.H. Chemistry, carcinogenicity and metabolism of 2-fluorenamine and related compounds, Adv. Cancer Res. 5, 331 (1958).

ENDOCRINE ASPECTS OF BREAST CANCER

O. H. Pearson

Department of Medicine
Case Western Reserve University
School of Medicine
Cleveland, Ohio

In 1896, a Scottish surgeon by the name of Beatson (1), reported the first therapeutic ovariectomies in two women with inoperable carcinoma of the breast. After study of the role of the ovaries on lactation in animals, he reasoned that removal of the ovaries might be helpful in the treatment of advanced, inoperable breast cancer. In two *premenopausal* women in whom this procedure was carried out, he described significant regression of the primary tumors in each case. Figures 1 and 2 illustrate the regression of a primary inoperable carcinoma of the breast which occurred following ovariectomy in a young woman.

Beatson's observation was amply confirmed at the turn of the century, and it was shown that 30 to 40 percent of premenopausal women with breast cancer obtained remissions following ovariectomy which lasted for about one year with subsequent reactivation of the disease. This therapeutic procedure was practiced only sporadically over the next 50 years, perhaps because it was not a curative procedure and was effective in only about one-third of the patients.

In the 1940's, when the gonadal hormones, estradiol and testosterone, became available for clinical use, it was shown that administration of these steroids could induce temporary regression of metastatic breast cancer in some patients, although occasionally these hormones seemed to accelerate the growth rate

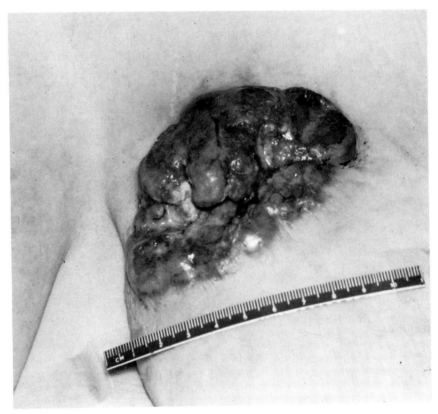

Fig. 1: Regression of a mammary cancer following ovariectomy. Before treatment.

of the tumors. Progesterone administration seemed to have little effect on tumor growth, but subsequently, when more potent derivatized progestins became available, remissions were induced in some patients with these steroids. In the 1950's, when cortisol became available, it was shown that administration of this hormone could induce temporary remission in some patients. With the availability of cortisol it became possible to remove the adrenal and pituitary glands from patients, and it was shown that these ablative procedures could induce significant regression of metastatic breast cancer in postmenopausal women as

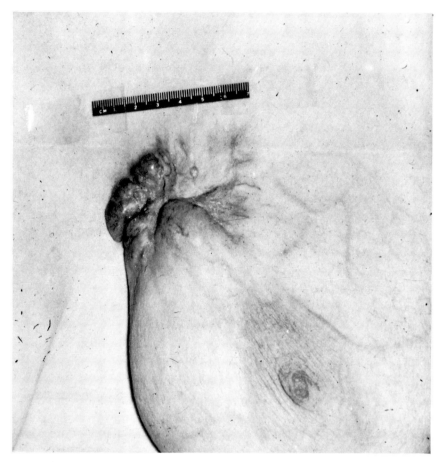

Fig. 2: Regression of a mammary cancer following ovariectomy. After treatment.

well as in those who had previously undergone ovari-ectomy. Figures 3 and 4 illustrate the regression of a primary inoperative, inflammatory carcinoma of the breast in a 70 year old woman following a hypophys-ectomy. Figure 5 demonstrates that metastatic lesions may also regress following endocrine treatment. Table 1 summarizes the author's approximation of the results which can be obtained from these endocrine manipula-tions.

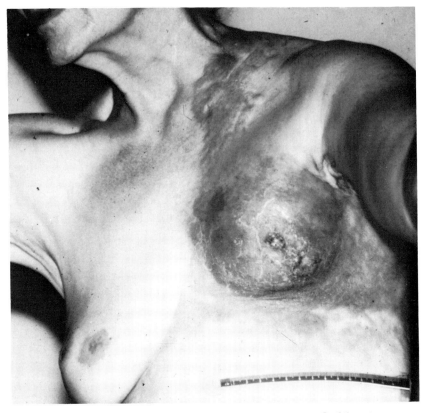

Fig. 3: Regression of a mammary cancer following
hypophysectomy. Before treatment.

     A number of hypotheses have been proposed to ex-
plain the empirical observations described above. One
hypothesis is that the growth of some malignant tumor
cells remains dependent upon hormonal function in the
host which is not unusual in kind or exaggerated in
rate. Thus, deprivation of essential hormones or interference with their action would result in cessation of growth and eventual elimination of some of the
cells, in the same manner that an endocrine target
organ undergoes atrophy when its essential hormone is
removed. To test this hypothesis, pilot studies were
carried out in patients which showed that, following

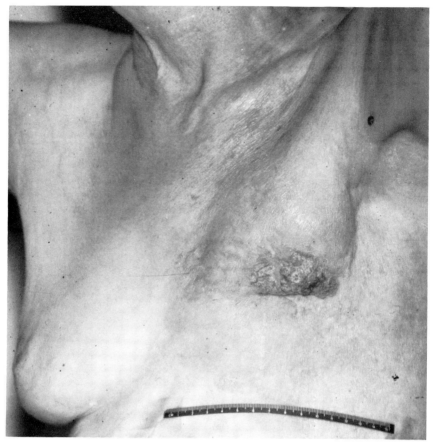

Fig. 4: Regression of a mammary cancer following hypophysectomy. After treatment.

ovariectomy-induced remissions, estrogen administration may reactivate tumor growth (19). Similar studies after an hypophysectomy-induced remission showed that estrogens failed to reactivate tumor growth suggesting that a pituitary factor was probably involved in the estrogenic stimulation of tumor growth (20). Because of the inherent difficulties of such studies in patients, an animal tumor model was sought which might provide the opportunity for more definitive

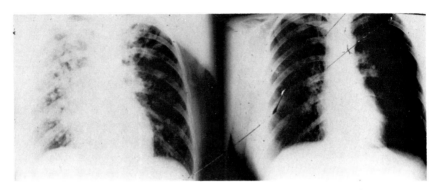

Fig. 5: Regression of pulmonary metastases from a mammary cancer following ovariectomy. Left, before treatment; right, after treatment.

studies of the endocrine factor, or factors, involved in the maintenance of mammary tumor growth.

Huggins and his coworkers (9) demonstrated that a single feeding of 7, 12-dimethylbenz-(a)-anthracene (DMBA) to 50 day old, female, Sprague-Dawley rats would produce breast cancer in 100 percent of the animals within 30 to 60 days. They also demonstrated that the majority of these cancers were hormone-dependent. We have used this model system for study of the endocrine factors involved in maintaining the growth of these tumors. In previously reported studies (23) it was shown that these cancers grow progressively in intact rats, and that animals die usually of inanition or infections. The tumors are adenocarcinomas which may invade local tissues but rarely, if ever, metastasize. Following oophorectomy and adrenalectomy or after hypophysectomy, the tumors regress completely and the animals live for several months without recurrence of the tumor. After an oophorectomy- and adrenalectomy-induced regression, estradiol benzoate administration in doses of 1 to 5 μg/day reactivates the growth of the tumor. When estradiol injections are discontinued, the tumors again regress. After a hypophysectomy-induced remission, estradiol benzoate injections failed to reactivate tumor growth even when cortisone and thyroxine

TABLE 1

AVERAGE INCIDENCE AND DURATION OF REMISSIONS
IN BREAST CANCER

Treatment	Incidence (per cent)	Duration (months)	Type of case
Hypophysectomy	40	18	Post-menopausal
Adrenalectomy	40	12	Post-menopausal
Oophorectomy	40	12	Pre-menopausal
Oestrogens	35	12	Post-menopausal
Provera	30	8	Post-menopausal
Androgens	20	6	Post-menopausal
Corticoids	30	3	Post-menopausal

injections were added to the estradiol. These results
indicated that the pituitary played a role in the estrogenic stimulation of rat mammary tumor growth and
resembled the results obtained in women with hormone-
responsive mammary cancer referred to above. Further
studies were undertaken in an attempt to define the
pituitary factor involved in the growth of the rat
mammary tumor.

Bovine growth hormone in doses of 2 to 4 mg/day
was administered to tumor bearing rats for 1 to 3 months
after partial regression of the tumors had been induced
by ovariectomy and adrenalectomy (21). There was no
evidence of stimulation of tumor growth in these animals. When ovine prolactin in doses of 0.5 to 2.0
mg/day was administered under similar circumstances,
there was prompt reactivation of tumor growth and the
tumors reached their original size in an average period of 18 days. When the prolactin injections were
discontinued, the tumors regressed to very small size
within 14 days. Ovine prolactin was administered to
rats whose mammary cancers had been induced to regress
following hypophysectomy. Reactivation of tumor growth
occurred within 16 days after starting prolactin injections, and the tumors regressed promptly when prolactin was discontinued. Estradiol benzoate injections,

5 μg per day for 39 days, failed to reactivate tumor
growth in these animals. Finally, ovine prolactin was
administered to rats whose mammary tumors had regressed
after ovariectomy, adrenalectomy and hypophysectomy.
Prolactin induced reactivation of tumor growth in all
of these animals. These results suggested that DMBA-
induced rat mammary carcinoma is prolactin-dependent,
and that the effects of estradiol on tumor growth might
be mediated through effects on pituitary prolactin secretion.

A radioimmunoassay for rat prolactin was developed
in order to study the effects of estradiol on prolactin
secretion (14). Serum prolactin levels were found to
fluctuate during the estrus cycle with a surge of prolactin secretion occurring just prior to ovulation.
Following ovariectomy and adrenalectomy, serum prolactin levels fell to about 50 percent of the diestrus
levels and there was no surge of prolactin secretion
such as occurs during the estrus cycle. After a single
injection of estradiol benzoate to an ovariectomized
rat, there was a 2 to 3 fold rise in serum prolactin
levels within 24 to 36 hours. Male rats have low
serum prolactin levels which show little fluctuation
from day to day. Daily administration of estradiol to
male rats produced a 3 to 4 fold rise in serum prolactin levels which was maintained. These observations
indicate that estradiol is an important regulator of
pituitary prolactin secretion in the rat and that the
surge in prolactin secretion which occurs at the time
of estrus is probably controlled by circulating estrogen levels.

Serum prolactin levels were measured in female
rats bearing DMBA-induced mammary cancers before and
after ovariectomy-adrenalectomy and after estradiol
administration (22). There was a good correlation between serum prolactin levels and the growth of the
mammary tumors. Thus, after ovariectomy-adrenalectomy
mammary tumors regressed in size and serum prolactin
levels fell, whereas, after estradiol administration
tumors grew in size and serum prolactin levels rose.
These observations are consistent with the concept

that ovariectomy-adrenalectomy induced regression of
rat mammary cancer is related to reduction in serum
prolactin levels, and that estradiol-induced reactivation of mammary tumor growth is related to rising serum
prolactin levels.

It has been demonstrated that certain tranquilizing drugs, such as the phenothiazines, induce mammotrophic and lactogenic effects in animals and man (12).
Using a radioimmunoassay for rat prolactin, we have
shown that a single injection of 4 mg of perphenazine
to a female rat produced a 10 fold rise in serum prolactin within one hour with a return toward control
levels within 24 hours (21). Daily administration of
perphenazine induced a sustained rise in serum prolactin levels. Perphenazine was administered daily to
DMBA-fed rats to determine whether this drug would
influence the development and rate of growth of mammary
tumors. It was found that the number and size of the
tumors in the perphenazine-treated animals far exceeded
those of the control rats. Perphenazine was also given
to DMBA-fed rats who underwent ovariectomy and adrenalectomy 6 days after feeding DMBA. After 5 months of
treatment with perphenazine, 7 of 15 rats developed
mammary cancers, whereas none of 11 control rats receiving saline injections developed palpable tumors.
These observations provide further evidence for the
importance of prolactin in maintaining the growth of
DMBA-induced rat mammary cancer.

Rabbit antiserum to purified rat prolactin was
administered to rats bearing DMBA-induced mammary cancers in order to assess possible inhibitory effects on
mammary tumor growth (2). Of 10 rats so treated, all
mammary tumors regressed in 5 animals, and in the other
5 rats some tumors regressed, some remained stable and
a few continued to grow. Inhibition of tumor growth
by prolactin antiserum was significantly greater than
in a control group of rats which received normal rabbit
serum. Estrus cycles continued to occur in these rats.
These observations provided further evidence for the
prolactin-dependence of DMBA-induced rat mammary cancer.

Estradiol benzoate in doses of 25 to 500 µg per day was administered to intact female rats bearing DMBA-induced mammary cancers (22). In each case estradiol induced regression of the rat mammary cancers. Serum prolactin levels rose progressively during estradiol treatment reaching 2 to 4 times the pre-treatment levels. It is apparent from these studies that the paradoxical effect of large doses of estrogen of causing regression of mammary cancer cannot be explained by suppression of pituitary prolactin secretion.

The possibility that the tumor-inhibiting effect of larger doses of estrogen might be due to a blocking of the peripheral action of prolactin on tumor growth has been examined in the following work, the results of which are as yet preliminary. Female rats bearing DMBA-induced mammary cancers underwent ovariectomy. When partial regression of the mammary tumors had occurred, perphenazine, 1 mg daily, was injected subcutaneously. When regrowth of the mammary cancers was established as a result of perphenazine injections, estradiol benzoate, 500 µg daily was added to the above regimen. During administration of estradiol striking regression of the mammary tumors occurred. The results of this experiment are consistent with the hypothesis that the tumor-inhibiting effects of large doses of estrogen are due to interference with the peripheral action of prolactin on tumor growth and not due to suppression of prolactin secretion.

Ergot alkaloids have been reported to inhibit lactation in the rat and Varavudhi *et al.* (26) suggested that the drug inhibits pituitary prolactin secretion. Administration of ergocornine to rats promptly lowers serum prolactin levels as determined by radioimmunoassay (16). The effects of this alkaloid were studied in rats bearing DMBA-induced mammary cancers. Ergocornine induced a 58% reduction of tumor area in seven rats after 20 days, and serum prolactin levels were markedly reduced. At this point estradiol was added to the regime, and the tumor size remained stable and serum prolactin levels increased somewhat. When perphenazine was substituted for the estradiol, serum prolactin levels rose and growth of the tumors resumed. In 5 control rats, tumors continued to grow and prolactin levels were normal. When ergocornine and estradiol were administered simultaneously, tumors regressed in size and serum prolactin levels fell. When ergocornine was discontinued, prolactin levels rose and tumor growth resumed. These observations lend further support to the concept of prolactin dependence of this rat mammary cancer.

The similarities between the DMBA-induced rat mammary cancer and hormone-responsive breast cancer in women suggest that the same endocrine factor may be oeprative in man as in rat, but this remains to be documented. During the past year, primate pituitary prolactin has been identified and isolated (7,17) and specific radioimmunoassays for the measurement of prolactin in human sera have been developed (10). Sensitive bioassays have also been developed (4) and there is a good correlation between bioassay and radioimmunoassay measurements of serum prolactin. Detailed studies of serum prolactin levels in breast cancer patients have not yet been reported, but preliminary studies suggest that basal serum prolactin levels are slightly higher than those in non-cancer patients or normal subjects.

Preliminary studies suggest that the regulation of prolactin secretion in man differs somewhat from that in the rat. No preovulatory surge in prolactin secretion has been noted during the menstrual cycle of women in contrast to the striking rise which occurs during the estrus cycle in rats (10). Estrogen administration induces a 2 to 3 fold rise in male subjects (5) as also occurs in the rat. In women, serum prolactin levels rise progressively during gestation (10), whereas in the rat prolactin levels rise only at the terminal phase of gestation. The role of estrogens in influencing prolactin secretion in man needs further exploration.

Phenothiazine drugs (thorazine) induce a prompt rise in serum prolactin levels in human subjects (13) as occurs in the rat. To my knowledge, ergot alkaloids

135

have not yet been tested in human subjects for possible effects on suppression of prolactin secretion. However, levodopa, a drug in common use for the treatment of Parkinson's disease, has been reported to suppress prolactin levels in normal subjects (8). This drug has also been reported to suppress the hypersecretion of prolactin in some women with galactorrhea and in addition suppresses the lactation (24). We have begun a pilot study of the effects of levodopa in selected patients with metastatic breast cancer and have observed regression of metastases in 2 of 7 patients after 2 months of treatment. Only partial suppression of serum prolactin was obtained with 0.5 gm levodopa given at 6 hour intervals. Further observations are needed to determine the extent of response which may be obtained by presumably suppressing prolactin secretion.

A recent report by Turkington and his colleagues (25) raises questions about the importance of prolactin in the growth of human breast cancer, however. These workers measured serum prolactin levels in 9 patients who had undergone pituitary stalk section for treatment of metastatic mammary carcinoma and found that serum prolactin levels were significantly elevated in 5 of these patients. Three of the five patients with elevated serum prolactin obtained objective remissions of their metastatic cancer. Thus, in these patients, increased prolactin secretion was not a deterrent to regression of their tumors. This may represent a different group of patients than those who improve after hypophysectomy.

One of the problems confronting the physician and the patient concerning endocrine treatment is that less than one half of the patients obtain benefit from the various hormonal manipulations which are available. Many studies have been carried out in an attempt to predict the hormone responsiveness of the tumors prior to the institution of therapy, but no simple, reliable test is yet available. Two approaches to this problem are worthy of mention. Jensen *et al* (11) have determined the presence or absence of a specific estrogen-binding protein in the cytosol of human mammary cancers obtained at biopsy. He has found that some mammary cancers have this estrogen-binding protein and others do not. He has correlated these findings with the response of the patient to endocrine ablative treatment and has found that when estrogen-binding protein is present in the tumor, the patient is likely to benefit from the treatment. McGuire and Julian (15) have performed similar studies of the DMBA-induced rat mammary cancer and have found that estrogen-binding protein is present in the hormone-dependent cancers but is undetectable in the hormone independent tumors. This approach seems to offer considerable promise in providing a practical method of predicting a therapeutic response. Frantz and Turkington (6) have reported specific binding of prolactin to the cell membrane fraction of normal mouse mammary tissue. It seems likely that, if prolactin directly stimulates mammary tumor growth, binding of this hormone to the cells membranes probably occurs. Studies are underway to determine whether hormone dependent mammary tumors bind prolactin whereas hormone independent tumors may not.

Knowledge of the endocrine factor, or factors, involved in the growth of human breast cancer should have significance in the optimal management of this disease. Although hypophysectomy appears to afford an optimal form of palliative endocrine therapy in those patients with hormone-responsive tumors, it is available only in certain medical centers with experienced personnel, and the procedure has not been widely applied. Specific chemotherapy which could accomplish the same results in a simpler manner would have distinct advantages. Not only could such therapy be more widely applied, but it could be instituted at an earlier phase of the disease. The reports of Nissen-Meyer (18) and of Cole (3) indicate that castration performed at the time of mastectomy is a more effective therapeutic procedure than where this therapy is reserved until metastases appear. The possibility that hypophysectomy or its medical equivalent might yield even more effective results is provocative. If prolactin should turn out to be the important endocrine factor in human breast cancer, it is conceivable that appropriate medical control of the secretion of this hormone might even have prophylactic value.

References

1. Beatson, G.T. On the treatment of inoperable cases of carcinoma of the mammae. Lancet 2, 104 (1896).

2. Butler, T. and Pearson, O.H. Regression of pro-lactin-dependent rat mammary carcinoma in response to antihormone treatment. Cancer Research 31, 817 (1971).

3. Cole, M.P. Suppression of ovarian function in primary breast cancer. In Prognostic Factors in Breast Cancer, A.P.M. Forrest and P.B. Kunkler (eds.), E. & S. Livingstone, Ltd., p. 146, 1968.

4. Frantz, A.G. and Kleinberg, D.L. Prolactin, evidence that it is separate from growth hormone in human blood. Science 170, 745 (1970).

5. Frantz, A.G. Human prolactin. Recent Prog. in Hormone Research (in press).

6. Frantz, W.L. and Turkington, R.W. The prolactin receptor: studies on its hormonal binding, chemical, and regulatory properties. Excerpta Medica, International Congress Series No. 256, p. 200, 1972.

7. Friesen, H. and Guyda, H. Biosynthesis of monkey growth hormone and prolactin in vitro. Endocrinology 88, 1353 (1971).

8. Friesen, H., personal communication.

9. Huggins, C., Grand, L.C. and Brillantes, F.P. Mammary cancer induced by a single feeding of polynuclear hydrocarbons and its suppression. Nature 189, 204 (1961).

10. Hwang, P., Guyda, H. and Friesen, H. A radioimmunoassay for human prolactin. Proc. Nat. Acad. Sci. U.S. 68, 1902 (1971).

11. Jensen, E.V., Block, G.E., Smith, S., Kyser, K. and DeSombre, E.R. Estrogen receptors and hormone dependency. In Estrogen Target Tissues and Neoplasia, T.L Dao (ed.), The University of Chicago Press, p. 23, 1972.

12. Khazan, N., Primo, Ch., Damon, A., Assael, M., Sulman, F.G. and Winnik, H.Z. The mammotrophic effects of tranquilizing drugs. Arch. Internat. Pharmacodyn. 136, 291 (1962).

13. Kleinberg, D.L., Wharton, R.N. and Frantz, A.G. Rapid release of prolactin in normal adults following chlorpromazine stimulation. 53rd Meeting of the Endocrine Society 88, A 126 (1971).

14. Llerena, L., Molina, A. and Pearson, O.H. Radioimmunoassay of rat prolactin. 51st Meeting of the Endocrine Society, p. 45, 1969.

15. McGuire, W.L. and Julian, J.A. Comparison of macromolecular binding of estradiol in hormone-dependent and hormone-independent rat mammary carcinoma. Cancer Research 31, 1440 (1971).

16. Nasr, H. and Pearson, O.H. Inhibition of prolactin secretion by ergot alkaloids. 53rd Meeting of the Endocrine Society 88, A 126 (1971).

17. Nasr, H., Pensky, J. and Pearson, O.H. Prolactin content of a pituitary tumor in Forbes Albright Syndrome. 52nd Meeting of the Endocrine Society, p. 129, 1970.

18. Nissen-Meyer, R. Suppression of ovarian function in primary breast cancer. In Prognostic Factors in Breast Cancer, A.P.M. Forrest and P.B. Kunkler (eds.), E. & S. Livingstone, Ltd, p. 139, 1968.

19. Pearson, O.H., West, C.D., Hollander, V.P. and Treves, N. Evaluation of endocrine therapy for advanced breast cancer. J.A.M.A. 154, 234 (1954).

20. Pearson, O.H. and Ray, B.S. Results of hypophysectomy in the treatment of metastatic mammary carcinoma. Cancer 12, 85 (1959).

21. Pearson, O.H., Llerena, O., Llerena, L., Molina, A and Butler, T. Prolactin-dependent rat mammary cancer: a model for man? Trans. Assn. Am. Physcians 32, 225 (1969).

22. Pearson, O.H., Molina, A., Butler, T., Llerena, L. and Nasr, H. Estrogens and prolactin in mammary cancer, In Estrogen Target Tissue and Neoplasia, T.L. Dao (ed.), Univ. of Chicago Press, p. 287, 1972.

23. Sterenthal, A., Dominguez, J.M., Weisman, C. and Pearson, O.H. Pituitary role in the estrogen dependency of experimental mammary cancer. Cancer Research 23, 481 (1963).

24. Turkington, R.W. Inhibition of prolactin and successful therapy of Forbes Albright Syndrome with L dopa. Proc. of Central Soc. for Clin. Research 44, 44 (1972).

25. Turkington, R.W., Underwood, L.E. and Van Wyk, J.J. Elevated serum prolactin levels after pituitary stalk section in man. New Eng. J. Med. 285, 707 (1971).

26. Varavudhi, P.B., Lobel, B.L. and Shelesnyak, M.C. Studies on the mechanism of nidation, effect of ergocornine in pregnant rats during experimentally induced delayed nidation. <u>J</u>. <u>Endocr</u>. <u>34</u>, 425 (1966).

IMMUNOTHERAPY OF CANCER

Herbert J. Rapp

Biology Branch
National Cancer Institute
National Institutes of Health
Bethesda, Maryland   20014

Immunotherapy has great appeal as a possible means of controlling cancer because it takes advantage of natural processes that are capable of absolute distinction between normal and cancer cells. Currently accepted methods of cancer treatment such as chemotherapy and x-irradiation, on the other hand, cause damage to both normal and cancer cells. Before immunotherapy can become a standard form of treatment for cancer in general, it will be necessary to find ways of increasing the potency of the immune response so that established tumors might be destroyed. This report deals with some recent advances in attempts to use the immune system to treat cancer in animals and humans. After a few general remarks about immunology and a brief discussion of the history and development of modern tumor immunology, some examples of approaches to cancer immunotherapy in animals and humans will be presented. Studies with a guinea pig model will be given in some detail, because they help in understanding how certain human tumors have been cured by an apparently immunologic process.

The Immune System-- Immunity may be thought of as a mixed response to substructures of molecules, foreign to the host, that gain access to the interior of the body. These antigens may be parts of bacterial cells, tumor cells, pollen grains, virus particles, or other agents. There are two major types of immune responses to an antigen. One of these responses is recognized by the appearance of serum proteins called antibodies or immunglobulins. These immunoglobulins have the ability to react with and bind the antigen to which the individual has been immunized. A homogeneous macromolecule made up of more than one functional group is multi-potent in terms of its antigenicity because each functional group can lead to the formation of antibody molecules that are unique for that group and no other on that molecule. Although antibody molecules have two or more sites capable of combining with a functional group on an antigen molecule, all of the sites on a given antibody molecule recognize only one particular type of functional group.

The other major immune response is recognized by the appearance of small lymphocytes that also have the capacity to react specifically with the antigen. The interaction of antigen and antibody, or antigen and sensitized lymphocytes, triggers certain reactions involving factors that are normally present in the host. For example, all normal individuals from fish to man contain a group of substances known as complement (28). In humans and guinea pigs this group of substances is made up of nine distinct proteins. Cells containing specific antibody on their surface activate the complement system and the culmination of this complicated sequence of reactions is the alteration of the permeability of the cell and, eventually, the death of the cell by osmotic lysis. Gram negative bacteria are particularly susceptible to the lytic action of antibody and complement and it is likely that these factors are responsible for preventing the progression of infection by certain organisms to a state that might produce pathology. There is evidence that tumor cells *in vivo* are destroyed by antibody and complement. There is no question that tumor cells are lysed *in vitro* by these reagents.

In the case of cell-mediated immunity (5) one of the recognized consequences of the interaction of antigen and specifically sensitized lymphocytes is the release from the lymphocytes of several factors. One of these called migration inhibition factor (MIF), has the capacity to prevent the migration of macrophages (7). As a consequence of this inhibition, macrophages accumulate at sites where lymphocytes have reacted with specific antigen and produce an inflammatory response-- a particularly intriguing aspect of the immune system for exploitation as a possible means of treating cancer.

History and Development of Tumor Immunology-- The history of tumor immunology dates back to the beginning of this century. At that time there were high hopes that an immunologic cancer cure was imminent. Those hopes were based on experiments in which animals, after being immunized with material derived from a transplantable tumor, were able to resist a challenge of living tumor tissue whereas the same dose of living tumor tissue given to an unimmunized animal grew progressively. In those days inbred animals were not available and it was eventually recognized that the ability of immunized animals to reject a tumor transplant was probably due to an immune response of the recipient to normal antigens of the donor. The recognition that rejection of those tumors was not tumor specific led to a generalized loss of interest in tumor immunology that lasted through the 1940's. These early experiments, however, provided the impetus for the development of inbred strains of mice and therefore, indirectly, gave birth to the science of transplantation immunology. When inbred mice became generally available a few brave individuals attempted to resurrect tumor immunology. Clearly, if the early experiments were repeated with inbred instead of random-bred mice, and if similar results were obtained, it would be difficult to ascribe the rejection of transplanted tumors by immunized mice to normal antigenic differences between donor and recipient.

An experiment that provided the link between early and modern tumor immunology was reported by Howard Andervont in 1937 (2). He injected living tumor cells into the skin of inbred mice and found that they produced a papule that increased in size for a few days and then regressed. The injection of these tumor cells into sites other than the skin produced progressively growing tumors. The tumor he used, however, was not derived from the strain of inbred mice he used in his experiments. The first report of an investigation in which the tumor and test animal were genetically compatible appeared in 1943 and was by Ludwik Gross (13). Gross produced sarcomas in inbred mice by the subcutaneous inoculation of methylcholanthrene. He then transplanted cells from these malignant tumors into the skin of normal inbred mice of the same strain in which the tumors arose. He found, as Andervont had, that tumor papules appeared, grew for a few days, and then regressed. After the skin tumors regressed he rechallenged the animals with cells from the same tumor and found that this time the tumors did not grow at all. The growth and regression of the first transplant was followed by the acquisition of the ability to reject a subsequent challenge. This experiment represents the beginning of modern tumor immunology.

Perhaps because most investigators were under the influence of the gloom and doom of the 1930's, the next significant paper did not appear until ten years later, in 1953. This was the work of Foley (11) who confirmed and extended Gross' observation. The tumors that Foley used were also induced by methylcholanthrene but the transplants grew progressively in the skin. To immunize the animals, therefore, he ligated the tumors and, after the tumors had resorbed, challenged the animals with the same tumor or another tumor that arose spontaneously in the same strain of mice. Animals immunized to the methylcholanthrene-induced tumor rejected this tumor but not the tumor which arose spontaneously. Foley's work introduced the concept that tumors resulting from different stimuli may not share the same transplantation antigens.

Four years later Prehn (27) published a paper which eventually led to a general reawakening of the possibility that tumor specific antigens may, after all, exist. He induced tumors in inbred mice by the administration of methylcholanthrene and then tested the question of whether immunization with a given tumor rendered the recipient capable of rejecting another tumor induced by the same chemical in the same strain of mice. His procedure was similar to Foley's but in addition Prehn showed that surgical excision of the transplants was an effective means of immunization. Prehn found that immunized mice were capable of suppressing the growth of transplants given at doses several times higher than that required to produce progressive growth in unimmunized mice. He presented evidence indicating that most of these chemically induced tumors possessed individually specific tumor transplantation antigens.

By 1960 the virologists were making important advances in tumor immunology. Habel (15) and Sjögren (32) established the fact that tumors induced by the polyoma virus contain tumor specific transplantation antigens. Since 1960 the rate of significant contributions to tumor immunology has greatly increased, due to the efforts of many investigators including Old (26), Law (20), Klein (18), Mathe (23), Baldwin (3), Morton (25), and Weiss (35).

As a result of these investigations the following picture of tumor immunology has emerged.

Tumors induced by non-viral carcinogens usually have individually distinct transplantation antigens whereas all tumors induced by a given virus share the same transplantation antigens. There are several types of antigens in or on tumor cells that are not detectable in normal cells. They may be located in the nucleus, the cytoplasm or on the surface of the tumor cell. As in the histo-compatibility systems the major mechanism of rejection is cell-mediated; that is, due to small lymphocytes specifically sensitized to tumor specific transplantation antigens. Anti-tumor immunity is characterized by a threshold. Thus, one can usually find a challenge dose high enough to overcome tumor immunity so that progressively growing tumors can be produced in spite of demonstrable tumor immunity. Antigens located inside tumor cells may be useful diagnostically; they are not known to influence transplantation rejection. Most tumor immunologists use transplants in their studies. There

is increasing evidence, however, for the existence of
tumor specific antigens on tumors arising in the primary host and for host recognition and reaction to
these antigens. A paradox of tumor immunity is that
tumors can grow progressively in the face of an unequivocal immune response to them. One explanation
for this observation is based on the evidence that
certain antibodies that react with tumors, called en-
hancing or blocking antibodies, may coat the cells
and thereby prevent cell-mediated immune processes
from killing the tumor (16). Individuals whose immune
systems are suppressed are at a greater risk of developing certain neoplasms than are those whose immune systems are intact. Until recently it was generally believed that all tumors contain unique antigens that are not present on normal tissues. Recently,
however several investigators have expressed some
doubts about this credo. For example, it has been
observed that antigens which were thought to be unique
to tumors could be demonstrated in normal fetal tissue
and, at low concentration, even in adult tissues (21).
Tumors may contain antigens that are not normally
found in the affected tissue or organ but may be
found normally in other organs. Another possibility
is that the carcinogenic process may lead to an auto-
immune response to normal organ specific antigens and
under certain conditions those antigens may appear
to be tumor specific. At present, therefore, there
is no unequivocal evidence for the existence of an
antigen on any tumor cell that is absolutely required
for the maintenance of the neoplastic state of that
cell and that is totally absent in any other normal
cell of the tumor-bearing host. Some investigators
have referred to these presumed tumor-specific antigens as "time and place antigens" (34). On the practical side, however, these "time and place antigens,"
although perhaps not strictly tumor specific, may be
useful in studies aimed at the etiology, prevention,
diagnosis, and therapy of cancer. At least in animal
models, and with some human neoplasms, immunotherapy
of cancer is a reality and it is, therefore, a worth-
while goal of immunologists to establish optimal conditions for cancer immunotherapy.

Cancer Prevention Versus Cancer Therapy-- Most of the evidence for the existence of tumor-specific transplantation antigens has come from prevention models like those already described. In the prevention models normal animals are first immunized to the tumor and then challenged with living tumor cells. While this kind of model provides strong evidence for the existence of tumor-specific antigens and a rational basis for immunotherapy, it is not directly applicable to the problem of reversing an established tumor. The prevention model is applicable for example to the prophylaxis of virus induced tumors. No one, however, has yet unequivocally identified an infectious agent that causes human cancer. Until, and even when, such agents are identified it is difficult to see how a safe and effective anti-cancer vaccine could be developed. The clinician is left then with the problem of finding ways to bring about the regression of established tumors.

There are two major approaches to cancer immunotherapy--specific and nonspecific. In the specific approach individuals with tumors are treated either by active immunization with material derived from tumor or by adoptive (passive) immunization, a procedure whereby sensitized lymphocytes, antibodies or both are transferred from an appropriately immunized donor to the recipient with the tumor. In the nonspecific approach agents that cause a generalized increase of immunity are administered to individuals with tumors. One of these agents is the BCG (Bacillus Calmette-Guerin) strain of Mycobacterium bovis. This is an organism which is now attenuated but was originally identified as a causative agent of bovine tuberculosis. It is used in many countries, but not the United States, as a vaccine for the prevention of human tuberculosis. These non-specific agents may be administered directly into the tumor or at sites remote from the tumor. Nonspecific stimulation of immunity may be followed by a specific immune response against the tumor. The tumors used in any model may be primary or transplanted. These considerations are summarized in Table 1.

TABLE 1
APPROACHES TO CANCER IMMUNOTHERAPY

IMMUNIZATION		TUMOR	ANIMAL	REFERENCE
TYPE	METHOD			
Specific	Active	Primary	Rabbit	8
		Transplant	Mouse Guinea pig Rat	22,31 19 33
	Passive	Primary	Mouse Rat Rabbit	10 1 9
		Transplant	Mouse Guinea pig	12 36
Non-specific	Direct	Primary	Human	17,24,30
		Transplant	Guinea pig	39
	Remote	Primary	Human	23
		Transplant	Mouse	22

A Guinea Pig Model for Cancer Immunotherapy--
When we began our work with the guinea pig there was
(and there still is) good reason to believe that the
immunologic rejection of tumors is mediated mainly by
sensitized lymphocytes. We reasoned that if cell-
mediated tumor immunity is an important mechanism for
the control of tumor growth, then it made sense to use
the guinea pig to study the mechanism of immunologic
tumor suppression. Guinea pigs, like human beings, but
unlike the usually available laboratory animals, are

capable of developing vigorous and prolonged, cell-
mediated delayed cutaneous hypersentitivity reactions
characterized by the delayed appearance of erythema
and induration following intradermal challenge with
antigen. Our first goal was to demonstrate tumor-
specific immunity by the delayed skin reaction. This
was accomplished in the following way (29,6). Inbred
guinea pigs, designated strain-2, were given the water
soluble carcinogen, diethylnitrosamine, in their drinking water. The concentration of carcinogen in the
drinking water was just below the toxic dose. The carcinogen was administered daily and the animals were
examined at intervals for the presence of tumor. Each
animal that received this agent eventually developed
a highly metastatic liver cancer. The time required
for tumor induction varied from 4 to 12 months. Individual tumor lines were developed by intraperitoneal
transplantation of cells derived from several primary
cancers. The first of these, line 1, has been characterized as a well-differentiated adenocarcinoma.
Several individual tumor lines each derived from a
different primary cancer are now available. In most
of the work presented here lines 1, 7, and 10 were used.
Line 7 has been characterized as a carcinosarcoma and
line 10 as a hepatocellular carcinoma.

Since the first goal was to determine whether
tumor-specific immunity could be detected by the delayed cutaneous hypersensitivity (DCH) reaction, ascites
cells of the line 1 tumor were injected intradermally
into normal strain 2 guinea pigs. In a few days growing tumor papules appeared at the site of injection
and, just as Gross had found with the mouse sarcomas,
the papules increased in size for several days and
then began to regress. Injection of tumor cells in-
tramuscularly on intraperitoneally produced fatal,
metastatic disease. After the skin tumors regressed,
the animals were challenged intradermally with living
line 1 tumor cells. The following day there were typical DCH reactions at the challenge sites. In unimmunized animals, the intradermal challenge produced no
DCH reactions and 7 days later there were tumor pap-

ules growing in the skin. At this time there was almost complete inhibition of tumor growth in the immunized animals. Animals immunized to line 1 tumor by
the growth and regression method developed systemic
immunity; that is, they were able to suppress the
growth of tumor cells administered at sites other than
the skin. This observation permitted us to devise experiments to test the efficacy of cancer immunotherapy.
The first treatment model to be described is somewhat
between prevention and therapy; the second is a true
therapy model.

An ideal model should fulfill three requirements,
1) tumor challenge must precede therapy, 2) an established tumor must be present before therapy is started,
and 3) metastases must be present before therapy is
started. The first model which fulfills the first but
not the second and third requirements and is intermed-
iate between prevention and therapy was set up in the
following way (19): Unimmunized strain-2 guinea pigs
received intramuscular injections of living line 1
tumor cells at a dose level that caused death of untreated animals in 60 to 90 days. Death was associated
with the appearance of pleural effusions following
metastasis to the lungs. Animals in the treatment
group received the first of three intradermal injections
of living line 1 tumor cells 5 days after the intramuscular challenge. The second dose was given one week
later and the third 2 weeks later. The first immunizing dose produced no delayed skin reaction and the papule increased in size at the same rate as in unimmunized animals without the intramuscular challenge.
The second and third immunizing doses produced delayed
skin reactions and there was no growth of tumor at the
injection sites in the skin. All 12 unimmunized animals were dead by 90 days while 5 of 12 immunized animals survived for more than a year and 4 remained tumor-
free for the rest of their lives. This experiment,
while, strictly speaking, not immunotherapy, demonstrated that it was possible to interfere with tumor
growth even if therapy is started after challenge; it
provided the impetus to devise more stringent tests of
the potency of cancer immunotherapy.

The next series of experiments provided the frame-
work for our current experimental efforts to study cancer immunotherapy. Preliminary experiments indicated
that tumor lines 1 and 7 did not share tumor-specific
transplantation antigens (41). Animals immunized to
line 1 were able to reject line 1 but not line 7 transplants and animals immunized to line 7 were able to
reject line 7 transplants but not line 1 transplants.
In the experiment, animals were immunized to line 1
tumor by the growth and regression method. Following
immunization the animals were challenged on the same
day at three separate sites. The first site received
living line 1 tumor cells, the second living line 7
tumor cells and the third a mixture of living line 1
and line 7 tumor cells. On the following day delayed
skin reactions were seen at the site containing line 1
cells alone and at the site containing the mixture.
No skin reaction developed at the site containing line
7 cells alone. During the next few days a growing
tumor papule developed at the site containing line 7
cells alone but no growth appeared at the site containing line 1 cells alone or at the site containing
the mixture of line 1 and line 7 (40). These results
were interpreted to mean that tumor suppression, at
least in part, involved components of the immune system which in themselves were not immunologically specific; that is, tumor cells that happen to be present
at a site where a delayed skin reaction is taking
place may be killed as "innocent bystanders." It was
also found that these animals developed specific immunity to line 7. The specific immunity may be responsible for maintaining the suppression of tumor growth.
    Attempts to establish the basis of this apparently
non-specific anti-tumor effect were based on the fact
that one of the main histologic features of delayed
skin reactions is the accumulation of large numbers
of mononuclear cells (presumably macrophages) at the
site of the reaction. Accordingly, peritoneal exudate
cells were obtained from a normal unimmunized strain-2
guinea pig, and macrophages separated from other cells
were injected into the skin of the same animal from

which the cells were taken. Six hours after the injection, erythema was present at the site. The growth
of line 7 tumor cells injected at the inflamed site
was suppressed (37). Inflammatory responses induced
by other agents were then tested for their inhibitory
effect on tumor growth. Tumor growth was suppressed
at sites of inflammation induced by turpentine, by
india ink, and by delayed skin reactions in response
to antigens unrelated to the tumor.

Migration inhibition factor (MIF) was also tested
for its ability to suppress tumor growth (4). MIF was
prepared *in vitro* with PPD, a purified protein derivative of tubercle bacilli, and MIF activity was assayed
by the measurement of inhibition of the migration of
macrophages from capillary tubes. A purified and con-
centrated fraction containing MIF was injected into
the skin of normal guinea pigs. Within 3 hours there
was a marked inflammatory reaction at the site of injection. Tumor cells injected into such a site did
not multiply. While it was clear that immunologically
non-specific components of the immune system exerted
an inhibitory effect on tumor growth, we also found,
from the results of other experiments, that this effect
was not potent enough to cause the regression of an
established tumor.

A search was begun for agents that produce stronger
inflammatory responses than those already tested. One
of the agents, BCG, was tested and found to be capable
of inducing regression not only of an established tumor
but early metastases as well. The series of experiments
that led to this result began when a new line of tumor
designated line 10 became available. Line 10 grew progressively in the skin but metastasized so rapidly to
the draining lymph node that it was not possible to immunize animals against this tumor by the methods previously used. Accordingly living line 10 tumor cells
were mixed with living BCG and the mixture injected
into the skin (38). There was no growth of tumor and
eventually animals developed specific systemic immunity
to line 10 tumor.

Experiments were performed to determine whether
BCG-induced tumor suppression was due to a direct cy-

totoxic effect by the BCG or whether a host response was required to eliminate the tumor. Present evidence indicates the latter to be the case. This evidence was derived from both *in vitro* and *in vivo* experiments. First, tumor cells in the presence of BCG incorporated tritiated thymidine to the same extent as tumor cells in the absence of BCG. In addition tumor cell viability was unaffected in the presence of BCG by the criterion of trypan blue dye exclusion. *In vivo* evidence that tumor cells are not directly affected by BCG was obtained in the following experiment. We knew from the work of others that the intravenous injection of BCG induces a state of immunosuppression so that the recipient is unable to develop a cell-mediated response to the BCG. Accordingly BCG was administered intravenously and a mixture of BCG and tumor cells was inoculated intradermally. Under these conditions tumor cells grew in the presence of BCG.

BCG was then tested for its capacity to eliminate established tumors. The results obtained suggested that this system might be a suitable model for study of immunotherapy. Normal strain-2 guinea pigs received intradermal injections of one million line 10 tumor cells. It was known from previous results that, by day 7 after challenge, this site would contain a tumor about 1 cm in diameter, weighing about 100 mg and that tumor cells would be present in the draining lymph node as a result of metastatic spread. On day 7, guinea pigs with tumors were treated in one of three ways. The tumors in one group of animals were treated by the intralesional injection of diluent, tumors were excised from a second group, and the third group received injections of living BCG into their tumors. Figure 1 shows a representative guinea pig 38 days after intralesional injection of diluent. The original transplant is growing and the lymph node metastasis is apparent. Figure 2 shows a guinea pig 38 days after the tumor was removed surgically; the original transplant has not returned but this animal has obvious lymph node metastasis. All animals in the first two groups eventually died of

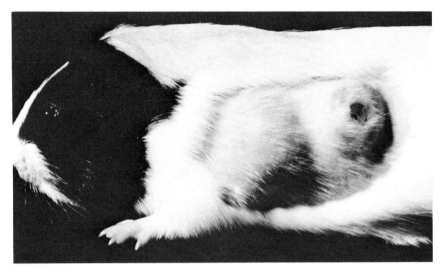

Fig. 1: Strain 2 guinea pig 38 days after intralesional injection of diluent given seven days after
intradermal transplantation of tumor.

metastic disease and there was no significant difference in the rate of death between the animals receiving
intratumor injections of diluent and the animals whose
tumors were excised. Figure 3 shows an animal 38 days
after injection of living BCG into the established
tumor. A scar, which eventually healed, is visible at
the injection site and there is no evidence of lymph
node metastasis. Most animals treated in this way
remained tumor-free for the rest of their lives. This
experiment was repeated using a 12 day interval between
challenge and treatment. On day 12, untreated tumors
weighed about 500 mg. While more than half the animals
treated with BCG on day 7 after challenge were permanently cured, this was true of only about 20% of the
animals treated 12 days after challenge. Histologic
examination of the node several days after injection
of BCG into the tumor transplants revealed the presence
of a large number of histiocytes in the nodes and a few
tumor cells that appeared to be degenerating (14).
Draining lymph nodes of cured animals eventually returned to normal appearance.

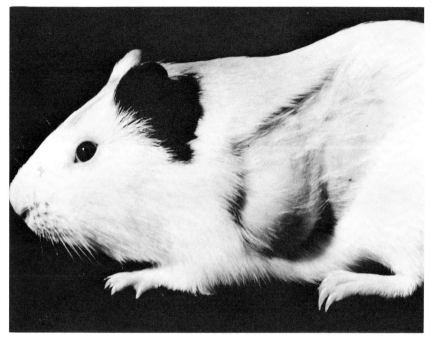

Fig. 2:   Strain 2 guinea pig 38 days after surgical
excision of seven day intradermal tumor transplant.

These experiments have suggested the following
hypothesis for the mechanism by which BCG produces this
remarkable anti-tumor effect. Following injection of
BCG into the tumor there are immunological responses
to BCG antigens. One of the responses is characterized
by the appearance of lymphocytes which have acquired
the immunologically specific ability to recognize and
react with BCG antigens. One of the consequences of
the interaction between these sensitized lymphocytes
and BCG antigens is the release of a soluble product
by the lymphocytes with the capacity to immobilize
macrophages or histiocytes. The BCG in our experiments
was injected directly into the tumor. The macrophages
or histiocytes that are immobilized by the MIF, therefore must, at least by chance, encounter tumor cells.
Although the BCG was injected into the tumor and not

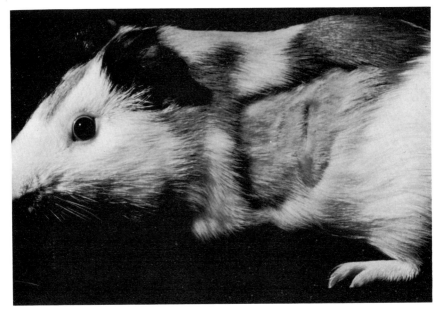

Fig. 3: Strain 2 guinea pig 38 days after intralesional injection of BCG given seven days after
intradermal transplantation of tumor.

into the lymph node, histological examination of the
node revealed the presence of acid-fast bacilli. This
means that the BCG-lymphocyte interaction with MIF release that takes place in the tumor transplant can
also take place in the lymph node. In some unknown
fashion, and apparently not requiring phagocytosis or
specific recognition of tumor antigens, the histiocytes
kill the tumor cells and perhaps a few host cells.
What happens next may be that the killed tumor cells,
by virtue of their destruction by the histiocytes, can
be processed by the immune system, resulting in the
appearance of lymphocytes specifically sensitized to
tumor antigens. These specifically sensitized lymphocytes can react directly with tumor antigen and either
kill the cells directly or, by releasing more MIF,
cause further influx of "angry" histiocytes. It is
possible, therefore, that the histiocytes serve at

least two purposes: 1) the immunologically non-specific destruction of tumor cells and 2) the mediation of a specific immune response leading to the appearance of lymphocytes specifically sensitized to tumor antigens.

Immunotherapy of Human Cancer-- I wish to summarize an immunotherapeutic treatment of human cancer being studied by Dr. Edmund Klein (17), who is head of the Dermatology Department of the Roswell Park Memorial Institute. He has been treating patients for more than 5 years by a method in which they are first sensitized to contact allergens such as dinitrochlorobenzene (DNCB) or 2,3-5 tri-ethylene iminobenzoquinine (TEIB). He then determines the concentration of allergen just below that necessary to produce a delayed cutaneous hypersensitivity reaction when applied to a normal area of the skin. This concentration, however, when applied to tumor sites elicits a delayed hypersensitivity reaction. It is not known why the tumor site is more responsive than the normal skin. In most cases after several such treatments Dr. Klein finds that the tumors go away and new skin grows over the site. Approximately 60 cases of skin carcinomas have been treated in this way and a high cure rate has been obtained with some patients remaining tumor free for 5 years. Preliminary work has also begun with a variety of pre-malignant and other malignant tumors.

There is a good chance that the basis of these findings of Dr. Klein is similar to the process described for the cure of the transplanted guinea pig hepatomas by BCG. Dr. Klein's results and ours raise the possibility that non-specific components of the immune system such as macrophages need to be activated in order to eliminate tumors; following the macrophage (histocyte) reaction, tumor specific immunity may be responsible for maintenance of the cure. Perhaps untreated tumors grow progressively even though they contain antigens that provoke a tumor specific immune response because the histocytes are not activated or if activated do not reach the tumor. Perhaps Dr. Klein's contact allergen treatment and our BCG treatment of animals are effective in cancer immunotherapy because these agents are administered directly into the tumor and at least in the case of BCG cause an accumulation of "angry" histiocytes at the tumor site. Studies are now in progress in the clinic and in the laboratory to determine whether the "angry" histiocyte response has general applicability to the treatment of cancer.

References

1. Alexander, P. Experiments with primary tumors and syngeneic tumor grafts. Progress in Exp. Tumor Res. 10, 22-71 (1968).

2. Andervont, H.B. The use of pure strain animals in studies of natural resistance to transplantable tumors. Pub. Health Rep. 52, 1885 (1937).

3. Baldwin, R.W. and Embleton, M.J. Tumor specific antigens in 2-acetylaminofluorene-induced rat hepatomas and related tumors. Israel J. Med. Sci. 7, 144 (1971).

4. Bernstein, I.D., Thor, D.E., Zbar, B. and Rapp, H.J. Tumor immunity: tumor suppression in vivo initiated by soluble products of specifically stimulated lymphocytes. Science 172, 729 (1971).

5. Chase, M.W. Delayed hypersensitivity. Med. Clin. N. Amer. 49, 1013 (1965).

6. Churchill, W.H., Jr., Rapp, H.J., Kronman, B.S. and Borsos, T. Detection of antigens of a new diethylnitrosamine-induced transplantable hepatoma by delayed hypersensitivity. J. Nat. Cancer Inst. 41, 13 (1968).

7. David, J.R. Delayed hypersensitivity in vitro: its mediation by cell-free substances formed by lymphoid cell-antigen interaction. Proc. Nat. Acad. Sci. U.S.A. 56, 72-77 (1966).

8. Evans, C.A., Gorman, L.R., Ito, Y. and Weiser, R.S. Anti-tumor immunity in the Shope papilloma-carcinoma complex of rabbits. I. Papilloma regression induced by homologous and autologous tissue vaccines. J. Nat. Cancer Inst. 29, 277 (1962).

9. Evans, C.A., Weiser, R.S. and Ito, Y. Antiviral and antitumor immunologic mechanisms operative in the Shope papilloma-carcinoma system. Cold Spring Harbor Symposia on Quantitative Biology XXVII, 453 (1962).

10. Fefer, A. Immunotherapy and chemotherapy of Moloney sarcoma-virus induced tumors in mice. Cancer Res. 29, 2177 (1969).

11. Foley, E.J. Antigenic properties of methylcholan-threne-induced tumors in mice of the strain of origin. Cancer Res. 13, 835 (1953).

12. Glynn, J.P., Halpern, B.L. and Fefer, A. An immunotherapeutic system for the treatment of a transplanted Moloney-virus induced lymphoma in mice. Cancer Res. 29, 515 (1969).

13. Gross, L. Intradermal immunization of C3H mice against a sarcoma that originated in an animal of the same line. Cancer Res. 3, 326 (1943).

14. Hanna, M.G., Zbar, B. and Rapp, H.J. Histopathology of tumor regression following intralesional injection of Mycobacterium bovis (BCG). II. Comparative effects of vaccinia virus, oxazolone and turpentine. J. Nat. Cancer Inst. 48, 1697 (1972).

15. Habel, K. Immunological determinants of polyoma virus oncogenesis. J. Exp. Med. 115, 181-193 (1962).

16. Hellström, I and Hellström, K.E. Colony inhibition studies on blocking and non-blocking serum

effects on cellular immunity to Moloney sarcomas. Int. J. Cancer 5, 195 (1970).

17. Klein, E. Hypersensitivity reactions at tumor sites. Cancer Res. 29, 2351 (1969).

18. Klein, G., Sjögren, H.O., Klein, E. and Hellström, K.E. Demonstration of resistance against methyl-cholanthrene-induced sarcomas in the primary autochthonous host. Cancer Res. 20, 1561 (1960).

19. Kronman, B., Wepsic, H.T., Churchill, W.H., Jr. Zbar, B., Borsos, T. and Rapp, H.J. Immunotherapy of cancer: an experimental model in syngeneic guinea pigs. Science 168, 257 (1970).

20. Law, L.W. Studies of thymic function with empha-sis on the role of the thymus in oncogenesis. Cancer Res. 26, 551 (1966).

21. Martin, F. and Martin, M.S. Radioimmunoassay of carcinoembryonic antigen in extracts of human colon and stomach. Int. J. Cancer 9, 641 (1971).

22. Mathe, G. Immunotherapie active de la leucemie L1210 appliquee apres la greffe tumorale. Revue Fraincaise d'Etudes Cliniques et Biologiques 13 881-883 (1968).

23. Mathe, G., Amiel, J.L., Schwarzenberg, L., Schneider, M., Cattan, A., Schlumberger, J.R., Hayat, M. and de Vassal, F. Active immunotherapy for acute lymphoblastic leukaemia. Lancet 1, 697 (1969).

24. Morton, D.L., Eilber, F.R., Malmgren, R.A. and Wood, W.C. Immunological factors which influence response to immunotherapy in malignant melanoma. Surgery 68, 158 (1970).

25. Morton, D.L., Miller, G.F. and Wood, D.A. Demon-stration of tumor specific immunity against anti-

gens unrelated to the mammary tumor virus in spontaneous mammary adenocarcinomas. J. Nat. Cancer Inst. 42, 289 (1969).

26. Old, L.J., Boyse, E.A., Clarke, D.A. and Carswell, E.A. Antigenic properties of chemically induced tumors. Ann. N.Y. Acad. Sci. 101, 80 (1962).

27. Prehn, R.T. and Main, J.M. Immunity to methylcholanthrene induced sarcomas. J. Nat. Cancer Inst. 18, 769 (1957).

28. Rapp, H.J. and Borsos, T. Molecular Basis of Complement Action. N.Y., Appleton-Century-Crofts, 1970.

29. Rapp, H.J., Churchill, W.H., Jr., Kronman, B.S., Rolley, R.T., Hammond, W.G. and Borsos, T. Antigenicity of a new diethylnitrosamine-induced transplantable guinea pig hepatoma: pathology and formation of ascites variant. J. Nat. Cancer Inst. 41, 1 (1968).

30. Ratner, A.C., Waldorf, D.S. and Van Scott, E.J. Alterations of lesions of mycosis fungoides lymphoma by direct imposition of delayed hypersensitivity reactions. Cancer 21, 83 (1968).

31. Slemmer, G. Effects of immunity on mouse mammary cancer. In Oncology 1970, Volume 2: Experimental cancer therapy (Clark R.L., Cumley, R.W., McKay, J.E., Copeland, M.M., eds.). Chicago, Yearbook Medical Publishers, 1971, pp. 483-494.

32. Sjögren, H.O. Studies on specific transplantation resistance to polyoma-virus-induced tumors. III. Transplantation resistance to genetically compatible polyoma tumors induced by polyoma tumor homografts. J. Nat. Cancer Inst. 32, 645-659 (1964).

33. Takeda, K., Kikuchi, Y., Yamawaki, S., Ueda, T. and Yoshiki, T. Treatment of artificial metastases of methylcholanthrene-induced rat sarcomas by autoimmunization of the autochthonous hosts. Cancer Res. 28, 2149 (1968).

34. Weiss, D.W. Perspectives of host-tumor relationships. Israel J. Med. Sci. 7, 1 (1971).

35. Weiss, D.W., Faulkin, L.J., Jr. and DeOme, K.B. Acquisition of heightened resistance and susceptibility to spontaneous mouse mammary carcinomas in the original host. Cancer Res. 24, 732 (1964).

36. Wepsic, H.T., Kronman, B.S., Zbar, B., Borsos, T. and Rapp, H.J. Immunotherapy of an intramuscular tumor in strain-2 guinea pigs: prevention of tumor growth by intradermal immunization and by systemic transfer of tumor immunity. J. Nat. Cancer Inst. 45, 377 (1970).

37. Zbar, B., Bernstein, I.D. and Rapp, H.J. Suppression of tumor growth by peritoneal exudate macrophages from unimmunized strain-2 guinea pigs. Proc. Amer. Assn. Cancer Res. 11, 87 (1970).

38. Zbar, B., Bernstein, I.D. and Rapp, H.J. Suppression of tumor growth at the site of infection with living Bacillus Calmette-Guerin. J. Nat. Cancer Inst. 46, 831 (1971).

39. Zbar, B. and Tanaka, T. Immunotherapy of cancer: regression of tumors after intralesional injection of living Mycobacterium bovis. Science 172, 271 (1971).

40. Zbar, B., Wepsic, H.T., Borsos, T. and Rapp, H.J. Tumor-graft rejection in syngeneic guinea pigs: evidence for a two-step mechanism. J. Nat. Cancer Inst. 43, 833 (1969).

41. Zbar, B., Wepsic, H.T., Rapp, H.J., Borsos, T., Kronman, B.S. and Churchill, W.H., Jr. Antigenic specificity of hepatomas induced in strain-2 guinea pigs by diethylnitrosamine. J. Nat. Cancer Inst. 43, 833 (1969).

CANCER CHEMOTHERAPY: CURRENT CONCEPTS AND RESULTS

Philip S. Schein

Medicine Branch
National Cancer Institute
National Institutes of Health
Bethesda, Maryland   20014

The field of cancer chemotherapy has, for many
years, been a stepchild of the medical community.
Negative attitudes can be traced to the relative in-
effectiveness and toxicity of drug treatment in the
past, combined with the basic nature of the disease;
many physicians have great difficulty dealing with
the psychologic burden that accompanies the responsi-
bility for the care of patients with cancer.

During the last five years, attitudes have
changed, albeit reluctantly, and the field of medical
oncology has rapidly emerged into a legitimate sub-
specialty of internal medicine. This has come about
partly because of the obvious need for physicians who
have specialized training in the management of cancer
patients, but also in recognition of the many advances
that have developed in the field of drug treatment.

In this review, I will outline many of the areas
in which chemotherapy has made notable progress and I
will use these selected examples as illustrations of
prevalent concepts and principles of treatment. In
addition, I will offer possible explanations for those
instances in which current therapy has made a lesser
contribution, particularly in the treatment of the
slower growing solid tumors.

There are major difficulties involved in the
identification of potential new clinical anticancer

agents. At the present time, the most active approach
to the selection of new drugs is largely empirical and
relies on the use of rodent tumor screens that have
shown a significant order of prediction for drug effectiveness in man (40,56). While one might have
hoped for a more direct method of identification, it
is acknowledged that the exact biochemical mechanisms
by which chemotherapeutic agents exert their antitumor
action have historically followed the demonstration of
clinical efficacy. Furthermore, there are many effective chemotherapeutic agents which have been in clinical use for years for which the prinicpal biochemical
mechanism of action, or explanation for selectivity
against a specific tumor awaits determination. However, two examples of a reasoned biochemical approach
to drug development or application merit discussion.
The recognition that certain experimental tumors
preferentially take up uracil compared to normal tissues led Hiedelberger and associates to synthesize a
compound which substituted a fluoride for hydrogen on
the fifth position of this pyrimidine (20). The resultant molecule, 5-fluorouracil inhibits the enzyme
thymidylate synthetase involved in the synthesis of
DNA, and is the present standard of drug therapy for
gastrointestinal malignancy.

The enzyme L-asparaginase has been shown to effectively deplete the peripheral body pool of the non-
essential amino acid L-asparagine and exploits the inability of some human leukemic cells to synthesize
sufficient quantities of this amino acid for their
metabolism and growth (19). However, such exploitable
differences in metabolism between normal and neoplastic
cells that allow for selective toxicity against the
tumor, have been few and difficult to demonstrate.
Particular patterns of biochemical action that have
been identified as having correlation with antitumor
activity, such as the inhibition of nucleic acid synthesis and alkylation have furnished important clues
for further drug synthesis and development. Nevertheless, the empirical approach to the identification
of new, effective therapies remains dominant while

awaiting advances from the laboratory, particularly from the field of molecular biology, which might allow for a more efficient method of prediction of clinical activity. At the same time, increased sophistication is being brought to the field of animal tumor screening. This has taken the form of testing for schedule dependency of drugs (53), and the use of animal tumors which have a reduced fraction of replicating cells and slow growth (40), kinetics that more closely resemble that of human solid tumors.

The present efforts to explain biochemical mechanisms of action have allowed a more rational approach to drug treatment. In particular, it is now possible to design a combination of drugs, each of which produces a different biochemical lesion, so as to attack multiple sites in biosynthetic pathways and/or inhibit several processes involved in maintenance and function of essential macromolecules. The common goal is to decrease the production and availability of a specific end product vital for tumor cell growth and replication. In this regard, three basic schemes have been described (Fig. 1):

  1. The inhibition of different enzymatic steps in a biochemical pathway leading to the production of an essential metabolite, has been designated sequential blockage as described by Potter (36). An example of this approach is the inhibition of de novo purine nucleotide synthesis by the combination of azaserine and 6-mercaptopurine.

  2. The simultaneous inhibition of parallel metabolic pathways involved in the synthesis of a common end product has been termed concurrent blockage by Elion (11). In the treatment of acute leukemia, use of 6-thioguanine and arabinosyl cytosine, which inhibit DNA synthesis by blocking the formation of a specific purine and pyrimidine respectively, in addition to inhibiting DNA polymerase, is representative of this form of inhibition.

  3. The most recent concept, that of complementary inhibition, envisions the selection of agents which produce biochemical lesions at different loci in the

169

synthesis of polymeric molecules (37). The use of alkylating agents to cross-link strands of DNA, in combination with antimetabolites which inhibit DNA synthesis and may prevent repair, serves as a possible example.

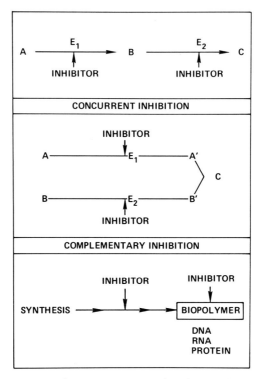

Fig. 1. Sequential Blockade

While this type of approach to the design of drug combinations is intellectually satisfying, it is recognized that such biochemical considerations are not always predictive of biologic synergism and in particular, they do not estimate the degree of depletion of the specific end product required for tumor cell destruction (37). It also assumes selective toxicity for the tumor tissue. Nevertheless, it is quite possible that many of the more promising drug combinations currently used in clinical cancer chemotherapy owe their effectiveness, in part, to such synergistic mechanisms.

In recent years, much attention in regard to bio-chemical mechanisms has been directed to the relation-ship of drug action to specific phases of the cell cycle, the series of events involved in individual cell replication. In brief, the cell cycle is composed of four phases as described in Figure 2. During the G_1 phase, the cell is basically in a resting state, though actively synthesizing RNA and protein. The total amount of time a cell remains in this phase is variable and may be quite prolonged if there is no stimulus to divide. As a result, the length of time spent in G_1 has, more than any other phase, a signifi-cant bearing on the rate of individual cell replica-tion. Once the cell has proceeded into the S phase, defined as that distinct period of the cell cycle de-voted to the synthesis of DNA, it is committed to complete the cycle. It progresses through the G_2 phase, which is concerned with RNA and protein synthe-sis, and the relatively short mitotic interval. The total time required to complete the cycle is termed the generation time.

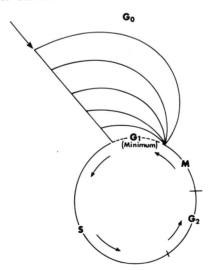

Fig. 2. The Cell Cycle (8)

171

An additional resting phase, G_0 or extended G_1, has also been defined, which represents an apparent state of non-proliferation, not necessarily associated with loss of replicative capacity.

Chem therapeutic agents can be classified as to their specificity of action in regard to the cell cycle as a whole, or to a specific phase of the cycle. An example of the latter category is the vinca alkaloids that act upon the mitotic spindle leading to arrest in metaphase of mitosis. Three major categories of compounds in regard to the cell cycle have been identified.

Group 1. S phase-specific agents such as arabinosyl cytosine and hydroxyurea, whose action is directed solely against cells actively synthesizing DNA. Group 2. S phase-specific but self-limited, including compounds such as 5-FU, methotrexate and 6-MP which are less effective therapeutically than Group I agents in experimental systems. The primary activity of this group is a blockage of DNA synthesis, but in addition, there may be inhibition of RNA and protein synthesis. It is postulated that this latter action slows the entry of cells into S from G_1 and thus protects the cell from the drug's principal lethal action in S phase. Group 3. Compounds such as the alkylating agents and nitrosoureas are considered non-cell cycle specific. The alkylating agents form complexes with DNA and can kill cells that are in all phases of the cell cycle. However, it is not known whether cells in G_1 are destroyed directly, or whether they are killed only when they attempt DNA replication, assuming that this occurs before there is an opportunity to repair damaged DNA.

This functional classification of biochemical action has gained much support because of its relevance to our present concepts of neoplastic cell growth, an understanding of which is basic to an appreciation of some of the major problems encountered in the treatment of solid tumors. While the initial stages of growth are exponential with a successive doubling in cell number, continued enlargement is

associated with a progressive increase in the doubling
time of the tumor. This apparent reduction of growth
results from an increase in cell death and lysis within the tumor (49), and to a decrease in the percentage
of cells in the actively proliferating growth fraction
(31). This phenomenon has been well described kinet-
ically by Tannock using a transplantable mouse mammary
tumor model (51). With continued enlargement, the
tumor gradually outgrows its sources of oxygen and
essential nutrients with resultant central necrosis –
a common observation in large human tumors. By dividing the large tumor into inner, middle and outer zones
with the respect to distance from the nutrient blood
vessel, it was possible to record a progressional decrease in the growth fraction, GF, in each of these
zones from 100 to 40 percent (Fig. 3). However, the
cell cycle time, TC, of individual replicating cells
was essentially identical for all zones. Thus the
major determinant of tumor growth was not the generation time of individual cells, but the total fraction
of cells actively dividing.

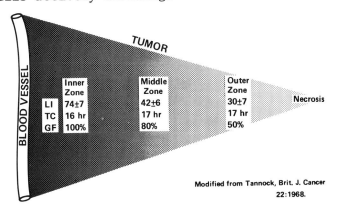

Fig. 3. Kinetic effect of vascular supply on mouse
mammary tumor.

Skipper and Zu-
brod have analyzed the current information on tumor
cell growth and advanced a conceptual model which des-
cribes three separate populations or proliferative

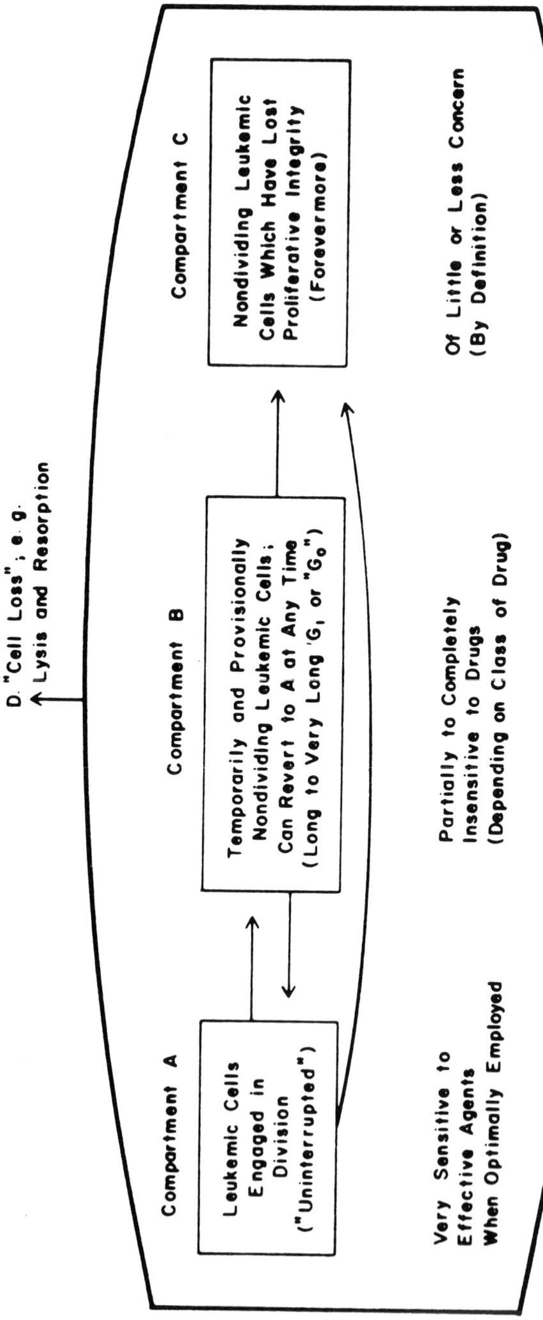
Compartment A
Leukemic Cells Engaged in Division ("Uninterrupted")
Very Sensitive to Effective Agents When Optimally Employed
Compartment B
Temporarily and Provisionally Nondividing Leukemic Cells; Can Revert to A at Any Time (Long to Very Long 'G1 or "G0")
Partially to Completely Insensitive to Drugs (Depending on Class of Drug)
Compartment C
Nondividing Leukemic Cells Which Have Lost Proliferative Integrity (Forevermore)
Of Little or Less Concern (By Definition)
D. "Cell Loss"; e.g. Lysis and Resorption

Figure 4

compartments of cells (Fig. 4)(47). Each of the compartments has a separate significance for chemotherapy.
Compartment A is composed of cells having a high
growth fraction and rapid cell turnover. Compartment
B is composed of a population of cells that are temporarily nondividing, or in terms of cell cycle kinetics, in a long G_1 or G_0 phase, but remain clonogenic.
The final compartment is composed of cells that have
permanently lost proliferative capacity but still
occupy volume in the tumor mass. It is the former
compartment of cells, A, to which therapy with currently available agents, in particular the cell cycle
specific anti-metabolites, can be directed most effectively. With increasing tumor size, the percent of
cells that leave compartment A and enter into a non-
proliferating state increases. This phenomenon is
presently considered to represent one of the major
limitations in solid tumor chemotherapy (43). Its
recognition has led to the use of combinations of
drugs that employ both cell cycle and non-cell cycle
specific agents, in an attempt to simultaneously deal
with both the dividing and non-dividing fractions of
cells within a tumor.

One notable exception to this general statement
of solid tumor kinetics is the Burkitt's tumor, an un-
differentiated malignant lymphoma, predominantly of
childhood. This tumor has been characterized as having an unusually large growth fraction and rapid cell
turnover (6). The natural history of Burkitt's tumor
is a rapidly fatal course in untreated cases. Ziegler
and his associates, using cyclophosphamide as a sole
therapy, have described a 100% complete remission rate
in patients with Stage I and II involvement where the
tumor is confined to a single, or two or more separate
facial masses. However, with more extensive tumor
spread, Stage III disease, the CR rate drops to 74%;
involvement of the central nervous system or bone
marrow limits the response to 28%. The induction of
a complete remission can be directly correlated with
a protracted disease free survival for the 20%
of patients who present with limited disease, and for

approximately 50% of all patients treated (59). It is quite probable that the high growth fraction of this tumor is a major factor for its responsiveness to chemotherapy. The need for early diagnosis and effective treatment of Burkitt's tumor, as in other forms of malignancy, is self-evident.

The quantitative aspects of tumor cell reduction by chemotherapy are best described by the cell-kill hypothesis as developed by Skipper and his associates. This concept is based on the following data derived from the L1210 mouse leukemia model (44,45).

1. Injection of a single leukemic cell into a BDF_1 mouse will ultimately lead to death of the animal. The implication is that for chemotherapy to be curative, it must destroy all tumor cells or reduce the cell number to a level where the host's immunologic surveillance might be effective.

2. With a larger innoculum of leukemic cells, a progressively shorter survival is recorded; the interval between innoculation of cells and death can be predicted by knowing the number of cells injected and the doubling time of the tumor. As an example, a single L1210 cell injected intraperitoneally kills in 19 days. This interval has been accounted for by a 2 day lag phase after transplantation, followed by 17 days of log phase growth. The L1210 system has a measured doubling time of approximately 12 hours, and assuming exponential growth, it can be calculated that the lethal number of cells at time of death was 10^9, or 9 logs. The time to death after the injection of 10^5 cells is a predictable 10 days (Fig. 5).

3. Using this model, it is possible to estimate the log cell kill and residual tumor cell number after a single treatment by extrapolating back from the prolongation in survival time. As demonstrated in Figure 6, an increase in life span of 2 days in this system would be equivalent to a 90% cell-kill which represents a 1 log reduction, in this case from 10^6 to 10^5. A course of treatment that will increase the life span of leukemic animals by 10 days can be calculated to have reduced the leukemic cell burden by

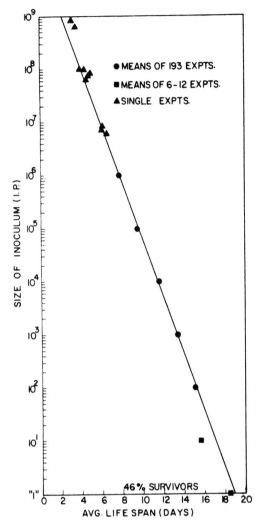

Fig. 5. Relationship between size of intraperitoneal inoculum and untreated host survival (44).

99.999% or 5 logs. This degree of cell kill will not cure the animal unless the initial tumor burden at time of treatment was 10^4 cells or less. As I will describe later, the principles of this model have been used clinically to determine the effectiveness of individual agents in childhood acute lymphocytic leukemia.

177

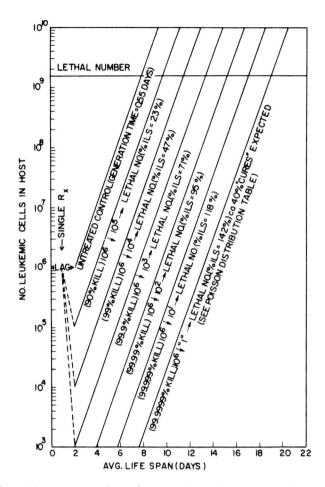

Fig. 6. Theoretical relationship between drug-induced kill of leukemic cells and percent increase in host life span (%ILS) after single dosage therapy; assumes no significant drug-induced lag phase (over that associated with transplantation) or increase in generation time of the surviving leukemic cells, no "compartments" inaccessible to the drug, and no drug-induced host lethality (44).

Intimately connected with the cell-kill concept has been skipper's recognition that a given dose of drug destroys a constant fraction of cells, not a fixed

number. This principle of fractional kill implies that
cell destruction by drugs follows first order kinetics,
a principle first described by microbiologists examining the effects of disinfectants on bacterial growth.
A course of treatment capable of reducing a cell population from 1,000,000 to 1000 cells, a 99.9% cell-kill
would also reduced a population of 1000 cells to one
cell.

The importance of the concepts of growth fraction
and fractional cell-kill to the effectiveness of chemotherapy has been most dramatically borne out by the
studies of Skipper with the L1210 leukemia using the
S-phase specific agent arabinosyl cytosine. The early
growth of the L1210 system is characterized by a
growth fraction of essentially 100% and a generation
time of 12 hours, of which 70% is spent in the synthesis of DNA (42). Pulses of ara-C were administered
every 3 hours for 24 hour periods in order to deliver
cytotoxic levels of the drug to successive cohorts of
leukemic cells entering into the chemotherapeutically
vulnerable period of DNA synthesis. The result was a
99.99% cell-kill (4 logs) with each successive course
of treatment, and cure of greater than 50% of animals
receiving repeated therapy at 4 day intervals (46).

While one can raise objections to several of the
assumptions of the cell-kill hypothesis, it has been
a useful model for organizing our thinking in the design and analysis of treatment programs. The implication of these concepts to the treatment of human
cancer is that eradication of a tumor will depend upon
the use of full doses of drugs to the tolerance of the
host, in an attempt to obtain the maximum cell-kill
potential of the compounds employed. This should be
done as early in the disease as possible when the total cell numbers are potentially within the therapeutic
limitations of a specific form of treatment, and before there is a significant reduction in the chemotherapeutically sensitive growth fraction. This latter
condition is seldom fulfilled in clinical oncology
where chemotherapy is commonly held in reserve until
such time as surgery and/or radiotherapy have been tried

and failed. In this situation, the chemotherapist is often asked to treat far advanced disease with his arsenal of agents which, though effective for palliation in many such instances, nevertheless have limited log kill potential and cannot be expected to significantly influence the course of disease at the time they are employed. This point was previously emphasized by the effect of advanced disease on the success in treatment of Burkitt's tumor.

We must also recognize that, at present, except for a few instances where a chemical or immunologic marker is available, we are plagued by our inability to detect and quantify so-called "early disease." Assuming that the tumor originated from a single transformed neoplastic cell and initial growth is exponential, a total of 27 doublings would be required to achieve a tumor nodule of 0.5 cm in diameter perhaps the realistic limits of routine physical examination and screening X-ray procedures (5). Such a nodule would contain approximately 10^8 cells with the full potential of metastatic lymphatic or blood stream spread prior to clinical recognition. With each additional doubling, the tumor diameter grows significantly so that at 35 doublings, a tumor 1 ft. in diameter might be produced, assuming continued exponential growth and no cell loss. Thus it may take only 7 to 8 cell doublings from diagnosis to death, giving a definite impression of rapid growth, although this interval represents only a segment of the continuum. It has been estimated that the total number of leukemic cells in a child with acute lymphocytic leukemia at time of diagnosis or frank relapse approximates 1×10^{12}, or 1 kg. of leukemic tumor tissue (15): thus the tumor burden in a patient with advanced and disseminated disease is enormous.

The principle of early treatment has been tested in a number of adult solid tumors, such as breast (14), lung (48) and colon (23), in the form of adjuvant drug therapy following surgery when the number of remaining tumor cells is presumably low. The results of these studies have largely been negative.

However, this is not at all surprising when one considers that these studies were carried out with single agents which have limited intrinsic activity against these tumors, and in some cases, at dose levels, which on experimental grounds, must be considered inadequate (43). The one possible exception in adult studies has been the use of 5-FU as an adjuvant after presumed "curative" resection of carcinoma of the colon (23). This ongoing study being carried out by the V.A. Surgical Adjuvant Group shows a 5 year survival of 57% and flattening of the curve for those patients randomized to 5-FU compared to 39% for controls (Fig. 7).

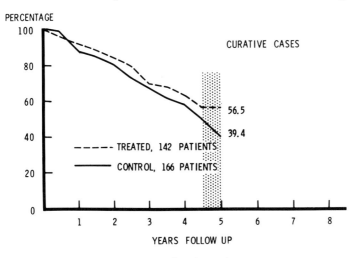

Fig. 7. Survival from randomization, 5-FU trial in carcinoma of the colon (23).

This data, though promising, must be regarded as preliminary until larger numbers of patients have reached the 5 year period of follow up. The most successful use of adjuvant chemotherapy has been in the treatment of Wilms' tumor, one of the most common neoplasms of infants and children. When actinomycin-D is administered at time of nephrectomy, followed by post-operative irradiation, not only are metastases prevented but the two year survival, tantamount to cure in this

181

disease, is increased to 60-90% compared to the 40%
obtained using surgery and radiation treatment alone
(13). In the presence of pulmonary metastases, previously regarded as essentially an incurable stage of
disease, the combination of actinomycin-D and palliative doses of radiotherapy have produced apparent
cures in 60% of cases. In a controlled trial, multiple
courses of actinomycin-D proved to be significantly
more effective than a single 5 day course (55). This
approach has now been extended to the treatment of
neuroblastoma (35), and rhabdomyosarcoma (54) in children. It is clear, that, as effective chemotherapeutic modalities for specific tumors are identified, one
of the major thrusts in future programs will be the
adjuvant approach in order to optimize the tumoricidal
potential of drug treatment.

Several additional major problem areas in chemotherapy that have recently been identified; recognition of each of these situations has eventually led
to particular innovative changes in both our overall
concepts and approach to treatment.

One of the significant obstacles of patient management in clinical chemotherapy is the difficulty in
estimating the neoplastic cell-kill and remaining cell
burden after each course of treatment. In solid tumors, the primary basis for the assessment of the
effectiveness of therapy has been of the measurement
of the uncorrected reduction in tumor volume or mass.
The dynamics involved within a solid tumor after treatment, are characterized in Figure 8. As suggested by
the curve, a 50-90% reduction in tumor cell volume,
clinically classified as a partial remission, may
represent as much as a 99.9% tumor cell-kill as determined by bioassay (43). This degree of cell-kill
is easily underestimated by simple measurement of
tumor size. The remaining viable neoplastic cells may
rapidly replace those that have been killed by treatment, while the dead cells are only slowly absorbed
and thus, for a period of time, will continue to con-
tribute to the tumor mass. The overall effect of
treatment on the size of a palpable tumor is much less

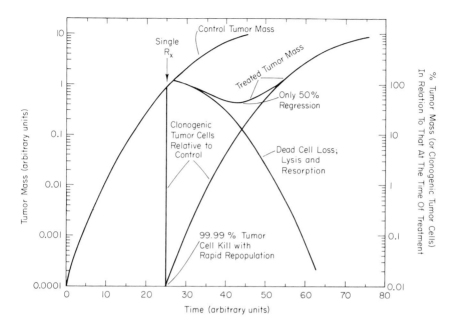

Fig. 8. Relationship of tumor volume to bioassay data on surviving tumor cells, as observed in solid animal tumors (43).

than one would have anticipated on the basis of fraction tumor cell-kill alone. The converse may also occur. If the initial size of the tumor is small at time of treatment, a 2-3 log cell-kill may be sufficient to produce a so-called complete remission, defined as total disappearance of clinically demonstrable disease. In this situation, measurement of tumor mass alone will overestimate the effectiveness of treatment While the drug has eliminated the top of the exponential tumor iceberg, there nevertheless remains many undetected logs of neoplastic cells that must be dealt with before cure can be effected. This difficulty in assessing response to therapy is not unique to solid tumors. In the treatment of acute leukemia, a reduction of 1 trillion leukemic cells, or a 4 log kill from the original 1×10^{12} estimated at relapse, will present as a complete remission (15). Nevertheless, 10^8 cells remain and retain the capacity to proliferate and exacerbate the disease.

In reaction to this problem, a major area of clinical investigation in oncology has been centered around the development of quantitative systems for estimating tumor cell burden (Table 1). The height of the abnor-

TABLE 1

USE OF BIOLOGICAL SUBSTANCES PRODUCED BY TUMORS
TO ASSESS PRESENCE AND EXTENT OF DISEASE

INDEX SUBSTANCE	TUMOR
Chorionic Gonadotrophin	Trophoblastic Disease
Immunoglobulins	Myeloma
Alpha Fetoprotein	Hepatoma
Placental Alkaline Phosphatase (Regan isoenzyme)	Lung, GI, Ovary
Tumor Specific Antigens (CEA)	Gastrointestinal
Ectopic Polypeptide Hormones	Lung, Kidney
Excessive Production Of Hormones Normally Produced By The Specific Tissue	Insulinoma, Carcinoid Adrenal Carcinoma
Catecholamine Metabolites	Neuroblastoma

mal globulin in patients with myeloma, the presence and titer of tumor specific antigens, the alpha fetoprotein produced by hepatomas, the Regan alkaline phosphatase isoenzyme, and ectopically produced polypeptide hormones are all currently being employed as indirect indices of tumor mass (58). The most successful application of this approach has been the quantitative measurement of chorionic gonadotrophin in patients with trophoblastic disease; hydatidiform mole, chorioadema destruens and choriocarcinoma. This assay has not only served as an important aid in diagnosis of these conditions, but has also allowed for an estimate of prognosis in individual cases. Hertz has shown that titers less than 1 million mouse uterine units/24 hour urine and institution of treatment within 4 months after onset of disease carries an excellent overall response rate and survival. The gestational trophoblastic tumors, as a group, have proved to be sensitive to a number of chemotherapeutic agents. Most studies have employed methotrexate combined, in more recent programs, with actinomycin-D, a drug that is effective in the face of MRX resistance. A complete remission status which for 1 year in this disease category correlates with a subsequent 5-10 year disease free survival which can be achieved in 50-90% of cases (26). Using the chorionic gonadotrophin titer, the chemotherapeutic management of these cases is markedly facilitated. It enables the physician to serially assess the effectiveness of treatment and chemically assay for the presence of neoplastic cells after clinical evidence of tumor has disappeared. It has also furnished a more sensitive guide for follow up of treated cases than is offered by routine physical measures.

The nature of the growth characteristics of human tumors requires that repeated courses of treatment be given over extended periods of time. This approach carries with it an increased risk for the development of drug toxicity, coupled with the fact that cancer chemotherapy agents, as a group, fail in varying degrees to discriminate efficiently between normal and target tissues. In the use of intensive combination chemotherapy, the clinician is frequently faced with the decision of timing a repeat course of treatment. A second cycle of therapy must be administered before there is regrowth of the tumor, while at the same time allowing a sufficient interval for the normal tissues, particularly the bone marrow, to recover from toxicity. An inappropriate delay can lead to an apparent failure of treatment.

It is fortunate that the killing effect of many of the standard chemotherapeutic agents can have a significant selectivity for malignant over normal host tissue. This statement is contrary to popular beliefs amongst physicians, particularly those who have limited experience using drugs in the treatment of neoplastic disease or who can only remember the early days in chemotherapy, when active agents were few and understanding of their use, limited. To illustrate this point of selectivity, I have selected an extreme example. The drug streptozotocin is an agent that produces a permanent diabetic state in laboratory animals through the specific destruction of the pancreatic beta cell (39). This pharmacologic property of streptozotocin has now been effectively exploited clinically in the treatment of malignant insulinoma, where a 70% functional (hormonal) and 40% objective response rate is being reported. However, streptozotocin has never produced clinically overt diabetes when administered to patients with non-insulin producing malignancies. This clearly demonstrates a specific sparing of the normal human pancreatic beta cell despite the administration of doses equal or in excess of that required for activity against some malignant beta cell tumors.

Experimentally, the selectivity of current antitumor agents has been examined by Bruce and co-workers using the spleen colony assay to quantitate survival of lymphoma vs. normal marrow stem cells of treated animals (4). Three distinct classes of chemotherapeutic agents could be defined with regard to the form of the dose-survival curve and relative sensitivity of the respective colony forming units (Table 2). Class I agents, irradiation and nitrogen mustard, which are non-cell cycle specific, produced an exponential survival curve with equal toxicity for normal hematologic and lymphoma colony-forming cells. Class II compounds, methotrexate, vinblastine and azaserine, which are cell cycle specific agents, produced an exponential cell-kill until a saturation value was reached. Lymphoma colony-forming units were significantly more sensitive to the action of these drugs than those of the normal bone marrow. The killing effect of the third class of compounds, including 5-fluorouracil, actinomycin-D and cyclophosphamide produced was exponential, again with much greater sensitivity of the lymphoma colony-forming cells as evidenced by a survival curve

TABLE 2

CLASSIFICATION OF CHEMOTHERAPEUTIC AGENTS BY DOSE-SURVIVAL
CURVES FOR LYMPHOMA AND MARROW COLONY FORMING CELLS

CLASS	AGENTS ASSIGNED	SURVIVAL CURES OBTAINED	DIFFERENTIAL SENSITIVITY BETWEEN MARROW AND LYMPHOMA CELLS	SUGGESTED ACTION AT CELLULAR LEVEL
I	γ Radiation Nitrogen Mustard BCNU	Exponential	None	Agents kill in all phases of cell cycle. (non-cell cycle dependent)
II	3H-Thymidine Vinblastine Amethopterin Azaserine	Decrease to constant saturation point at high doses	500 fold greater cell kill of lymphoma colony forming cells	Agents kill in only one phase of the cell cycle. Cells not entering this portion during treatment survive.
III	5-Fluorouracil Actinomycin D Cyclophosphamide	Exponential	10,000 fold greater cell kill of lymphoma colony forming cells	Agents active in several phases of the cell cycle but sensitivity strongly depends on fraction in proliferative state.

that was 6-10 times as steep as that for normal hematopoietic units. This differential activity against the
lymphoma cells by agents that depend on active proliferation, the Class II and III compounds, could be
correlated with the higher growth fraction of the tumor
compared to that of the normal hematopoietic stem cell.

Although dose-response relationships of current
drugs suggest greater antitumor activity at higher dose
levels, life-threatening toxicity has not been shown to
be a prerequisite for therapeutic response. Drug toxicity, in itself, can obscure the beneficial effect
obtained in solid tumors, lymphoma and chronic leukemias.
This has been well demonstrated for the use of 5-FU
in the treatment of colon-rectal cancer where the best
response rates have been correlated with the production
of a moderate, but not an advanced degree of leukopenia
(Fig. 9).

One definite exception to this general statement
is illustrated by the current therapeutic approach to
the treatment of acute myelogenous leukemia. The most
active regimens produce a near complete elimination of
bone marrow elements in an attempt to effectively reduce the leukemic clone. In doing so, it is hoped that
the marrow will subsequently be repopulated by the surviving normal hematopoietic stem cells. While awaiting
this response, the patient remains at risk from infection and hemorrhage for several weeks. This has
necessitated the development of the important sub-
specialty of supportive care in the field of medical
oncology. The development of measures to reduce the
patient's exposure to both exogenous and endogenous
microbial flora by the use of protective environments,
laminar flow rooms and antibiotic bowel sterilization
programs have been shown to lessen the number of serious infections during this highly vulnerable period
(41). The methodologic and immunologic advances in
the use of platelet transfusions have effectively reduced the threat of hemorrhage from thrombocytopenia
(57). The application of our present understanding
of uric acid metabolism and the development of allo-
purinol have dealt with the past problem of renal tub-
ular obstruction by urates, resulting from the rapid

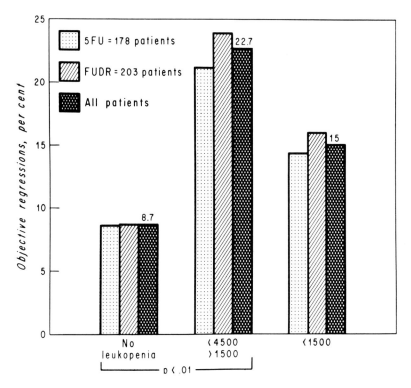

Fig. 9: Relationship of degree of toxicity to therapeutic effectiveness of the fluorinated pyrimidines
in colon-rectal cancer (32).

dissolution of leukemic and lymphomatous tissue. With
the use of these supportive measures, greater numbers
of patients with acute leukemia in particular, are
able to undergo the rigors of remission induction therapy. As a result, these developments in ancillary
care must be regarded as a contributory factor to the
improving response rates in these diseases.

The general problem of resistance to treatment in
cancer chemotherapy is extremely complex. In addition
to the difficulties imposed by the inherent features
of tumor cell growth previously described, schedule of
administration, pharmacologic barriers and various
forms of drug resistance have been identified.

It is now recognized that the schedule at which
a drug is given can markedly influence its therapeutic
index and that treatment with an effective chemotherapeutic agent may fail as a result of the use of a less
than optimal schedule of administration. In 1956,
Goldin demonstrated that methotrexate administered every 4 days was more effective against the L1210 leukemia than the same drug given daily (18). Subsequently,
a clinical trial of the effect of dose-schedule and
route of MTX for maintenance of complete remissions in
childhood leukemia was carried out. Patients were randomized to either daily oral treatment at 3 mg/m^2/day
or to a twice weekly intramuscular schedule at a dose
of 30 mg/m^2. The toxicity for the two programs per
unit time was comparable. However, the median duration
of remission for the intermittant MTX program was 1 year
compared to only 12 weeks for the daily schedule (38).
This study well illustrates the concept of "schedule
resistance" and emphasizes the importance of determining the most optimal treatment interval for specific
agents. In some instances, this may be as important a
consideration as choice of dose.

One of the major obstacles recognized in the treatment of acute lymphocytic leukemia of childhood has
been the failure of drugs to penetrate certain biological barriers and specific organis in sufficient cidal
concentration. From this has been developed the concept of "pharmacologic sanctuaries," of which the subarachnoid space is a principal example. Slightly over
50% of relapses in acute lymphocytic leukemia initially
take place in the form of meningeal involvement (2).
Leukemic cells lying within the subarachnoid space are
protected from exposure from high drug concentrations
by the relative exclusion of most clinically active
compounds by the blood-brain-barrier. Infiltration of
solid organs such as testicle, ovary and kidney represent additional areas of possible inadequate drug pen-
etration leaving viable cells that may exacerbate the
disease when therapy is withdrawn. Moreover, in this
milieu of low drug concentration, the situation is optimal for the development of drug resistance.

A variety of possible physiologic and biochemical mechanisms of drug resistance have been described in experimental tumor systems (Table 3). In general, the relative importance of each of these for human tumor cells remains speculative. An important area of clinical research in cancer chemotherapy involves the development of *in vitro* tests that will predict responsiveness of tumor cell lines of individual patients to specific drugs. This is essential, not only for a more direct basis for drug selection, but also to spare some patients the toxicity of, what is for their specific tumor, an ineffective therapy.

TABLE 3

RESISTANCE TO ANTICANCER DRUGS

Mechanism	Example
1. Insufficient drug uptake by the neoplastic cell	Methotrexate Daunomycin
2. Insufficient activation of drug	6-Mercaptopurine 5-Fluorouracil
3. Increased inactivation	Arabinosyl Cytosine
4. Increased concentration of a target enzyme	Methotrexate
5. Decreased requirement for a specific metabolic product	L-Asparaginase
6. Increased utilization of an alternative biochemical pathway (salvage)	Antimetabolites
7. Rapid repair of a drug induced lesion	Alkylating agents

One such *in vitro* system has been proposed for arabinosyl cytosine in acute myelogenous leukemia (50). Within the leukemic cell, this compound is activated by phosphorylation and inactivated by deamination. The ratio of the activities of the enzymes involved in these reactions has been shown to correlate well with an individual patient's response to treatment. Sequential measurements of these enzymes after repeated courses of therapy with arabinosyl cytosine demonstrated an increase in deaminating or inactivating activity in association with clinical refractoriness to further treatment.

Drug resistance, as in this latter illustration, may develop as a stepwise induction or may be related to a group of cells that are inherently resistant to the drug employed, irregardless of dose. In the latter situation, the use of additional effective drugs is essential since the single agent used alone will eventually select out this resistant cell line and, as a result, produce only a temporary response.

From this brief discussion of the general problem of resistance, we can now logically proceed to the clinical methods that have been developed to deal with these obstacles to drug treatment. The major effort has been the development of effective drug combinations which have been based on the following general principles:

1. The successful combined drug programs have used compounds which are individually active in the specific disease. It has become apparent that studies using agents, which by themselves have no significant clinical effect, often leads to increased toxicity with no therapeutic gain (33).

2. Drugs that act by different known mechanisms of action are selected in an attempt to achieve a degree of synergism and overcome potential problems of resistance.

3. Drug selection must take into account the dose-limiting toxicity of each compound chosen so as not to result in accumulative toxicity against a single organ system, such as the bone marrow. This has allowed for use of the individual drugs in full clinical dosage, a requirement for effectiveness in some combinations.

4. Intermittent schedules of 2 to 6 weeks have been used to allow for bone marrow recovery after intensive full does treatment. A second cycle of therapy is instituted before the tumor has regrown to the pretreatment level.

These principles are well illustrated by examining the developments that have taken place in the treatment of childhood acute lymphatic leukemia.

Following Farber's demonstration in 1947 that remission in acute lymphatic leukemia could be achieved with the folate-antagonist aminopterin, at least 12 individual compounds have been identified as having significant therapeutic activity in this disease (Table 4)(21). However, the length of complete remission produced by single agents has been shown to be relatively short, in the range of 1 to 2 months. Using the concepts developed in the L1210 model, one can extrapolate an estimate of the cell-kill produced by individual drugs based on the time to relapse from an unmaintained remission. Assuming that the average doubling time of leukemic cells is 4 days and that 10^{12} cells are present at time of exacerbation, these calculations suggest that single agents, such as vincristine or prednisone, effected only a 3-4 log reduction in leukemic cell burden to produce a complete remission status.

TABLE 4

DRUGS THAT INDUCE COMPLETE REMISSIONS IN
ACUTE LYMPHATIC LEUKEMIA

Agent	Percent Complete Remission
Prednisone	19–76
Vincristine	44–57
Methotrexate	22–31
6-Mercaptopurine	27–42
Daunomycin	33–50
Adriamycin	50
Cytosine Arabinoside	30
L-Asparaginase	30–67
Cyclophosphamide	3–76
Methyl-GAG	30
ICRF 159	25
BCNU	15

The next phase of development involved the study of combinations of remission inducing drugs in an attempt to demonstrate an additive or synergistic action. The result was an increase in the percentage of patients

achieving complete remission to the range of 80-90%
(Fig. 10)(12). The combination of vincristine and
prednisone has become the standard remission induction
regimen. It has largely been selected because of its
effectiveness, but also because neither compound is
significantly myelosuppressive, and the respective
dose-limiting toxicities of these two drugs differ.

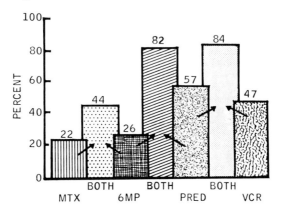

Fig. 10: Percent remission induction in acute lymphocyte leukemia by single agents and combinations (shown
in adjacent pairs)(12).

The concept of maintenance therapy developed
from the observation that additional drug treatment
would be required to prolong the complete remission
status. The remission induction agents, vincristine
and prednisone, proved unsatisfactory for this purpose,
and the first demonstration of the effectiveness of
this approach was the production of a 3-fold increased
duration in prednisone induced remissions by 6-mercap-
topurine (16).

Subsequently, a number of regimens, composed of
methotrexate consolidation and extended maintenance,
with and without reinduction therapy with vincristine
and prednisone, have been tested by the Acute Leukemia
Group B. These systematic clinical trials have resulted in an increase in the 5 year survival to approximately 25% (24).

Concurrent with this work, the Acute Leukemia Service of the National Cancer Institute has investigated the use of intensive 4 drug combinations as both a remission induction and consolidation therapy. The agents used have included vincristine, prednisone, 6-mercaptopurine, and methotrexate or cyclophosphamide which has given rise to the acronyms VAMP and POMP by which the combinations have been identified. The duration of unmaintained remission following these regimens, while prolonged, have unfortunately not significantly differed from those produced by the aforementioned programs, despite an estimated 10 log cell kill with the VAMP combination (15,22).

The next major advance in the treatment of acute lymphocytic leukemia has resulted from the recognition that the subarachnoid space is the initial site of relapse in slightly greater than 50% of cases. The St. Jude Children's Research Hospital designed an additional phase into their treatment program to deal with the problem of the central nervous system pharmacologic barrier. After initial remission induction and consolidation chemotherapy, children have received prophylactic cranial radiation of 2400R and 5 intrathecal doses of methotrexate. This is followed by maintenance drug therapy that is extended over a 2-3 year period. The results to date are quite encouraging. Seventy-one percent of all patients entered into the program, and 78% of those achieving an initial CR, have survived 2 years or more (2). Only 3 of the 30 patients who attained remission have developed CNS leukemia as the initial site of relapse. It is estimated that approximately 50% of these children may be alive without evidence of leukemia at 5 years.

The use of active immunotherapy at a point where leukemic cells have been reduced to small numbers by drug treatment, has great theoretical potential for elimination of the last remaining neoplastic cells. Mathe has employed BCG and/or allogenic leukemic cell immunization as a maintenance therapy after intensive induction and consolidation chemotherapy and CNS irradiation (29). This study demonstrated significant synergism between chemotherapy and immunotherapy with a projected extended disease free survival of 35%, compared to the relatively poor response for patients given no maintenance treatment (Fig. 11). Enthusiasm for this approach must be tempered with the knowledge that this very promising result has not as yet been confirmed in controlled trials, at other institutions.

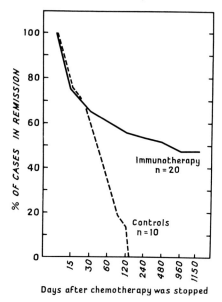

Fig. 11:   (29)

The chemotherapeutic approach to the treatment of lymphomas has made much progress during the past 5 years. This has resulted largely from the more effective use of established and recently developed active compounds in combinations, coupled with an increased sophistication in our understanding of the natural history of these disorders, in relationship to their histopathology. An additional factor has been the advent of more extensive staging procedures, particularly lymphangiography and more recently laparotomy. These have not only increased our insight into the modes and pattern of spread but has also re-emphasized the importance of extent of disease to the quality and length of response to treatment.

In the case of Hodgkin's disease, a number of different classes of antitumor agents have been demonstrated to be clinically active, including the alkylating agents, the vinca alkaloids, the methylhydrazine derivative procarbazine, the corticosteroids and the nitrosoureas (9,52). The overall response of Hodgkin's disease to single drug therapy varies from 40-75%. However, the rate of complete remission is considerably lower, in the range of 10-30%, with a median unmaintained duration of only 3 months. As can be seen in Table 5, several of these compounds including BCNU, vincristine and procarbazine have had clinical trials only in patients who have had extensive prior therapy, a factor that has been demonstrated to adversely affect the ability to obtain a complete remission. In terms of survival, patients treated with single agent therapy have, on the average, lived less than 2 years.

TABLE 5

HODGKIN'S DISEASE — SINGLE AGENT TREATMENT

Treatment	Percent Complete Remission	Percent Overall Response	Mean Duration of Remission No Maintenance (Months)	Mean Duration of Remission with Maintenance Therapy (Months)
Nitrogen Mustard	20	61	2.5	---
Cyclophosphamide	20	59	3.0	7.0
Vinblastine	27	64	3.0	6.5
Vincristine*	< 10	---	---	---
Procarbazine*	< 10	75	---	4.0
Prednisone*	< 5	---	---	---
BCNU*	< 5	55	---	5.0

*Patients had received extensive prior therapy.

In 1964, Drs. DeVita and Carbone, of the National Cancer Institute, developed a 4 drug combination protocol for Hodgkin's disease, which has become known as the MOPP program, as outlined in Figure 12. A total of 6 cycles of this combination were given, each of which was alternated with an intervening 2 week rest period. By 1967, 43 consecutive patients with predominantly Stage 4B disease had been entered onto the study (10). Thirty-five of the original 43 patients, or 81%, achieved a complete remission and were followed without further therapy. Of the complete remitters, 15 or 43% remain continuously free of disease. Twenty of the 35 complete responders have relapsed and have been retreated, and 9 are alive on maintenance therapy.

Drugs	Day 1	Day 8	Day 14	Day 28
Vincristine	1.4	1.4	Rest period	
Nitrogen mustard	6	6		
Procarbazine	100		→	
Prednisone[a]	40		→	

[a] Cycles 1 and 4 only.

Fig. 12: The MOPP program for advanced Hodgkin's disease.

Thus, approximately 70% of patients who had an initial complete response, are alive a minimum of 4 years. The median survival for either the complete responders or, the study as a whole, has not been reached but will exceed 5 years for the complete remission group, which represents a major advance over results with single agent therapy (Figure 13). The data comes into better perspective when one compares survival in advanced Hodgkin's disease with that in one of the so-called benign conditions common to medical practice, congestive heart failure. This malady has had, since Withering's introduction of the foxglove, the benefit of over 100 years of extensive drug development and treatment. Despite modern management, CHF remains a very

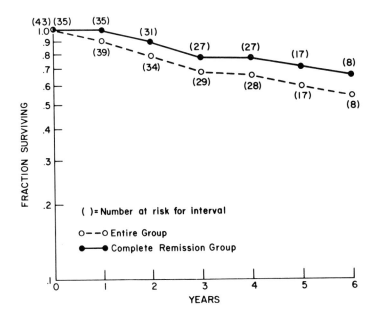

Fig. 13: Life table analysis of survival following combination chemotherapy.

lethal disease with a 5 year survival of only 38% for men (30).

The very promising results in advanced Hodgkin's disease have now been confirmed by a number of clinical trials at other institutions including a large British study (34). Several programs are now in progress incorporating various forms of maintenance treatment after MOPP or combining the separate modalities of combination chemotherapy and radiotherapy. Each of these approaches may be expected to further improve the duration of disease free survival.

A similar approach is now being taken in the treatment of lymphosarcoma. The results of single drug studies have demonstrated a response in approximately 60% of cases but with complete remission rates of only 10-15%. The median duration of maintained remissions have been in the range of 3-8 months (9,52).

In a program conducted at the National Cancer Institute, 35 consecutive patients with lymphocytic lymphoma, the vast majority with Stage IV or extra nodal disease, have been treated with a combination of cyclophosphamide, vincristine and prednisone (the CVP regimen) outlined in Figure 14. Cycles of therapy are administered every 3 weeks, usually on an outpatient

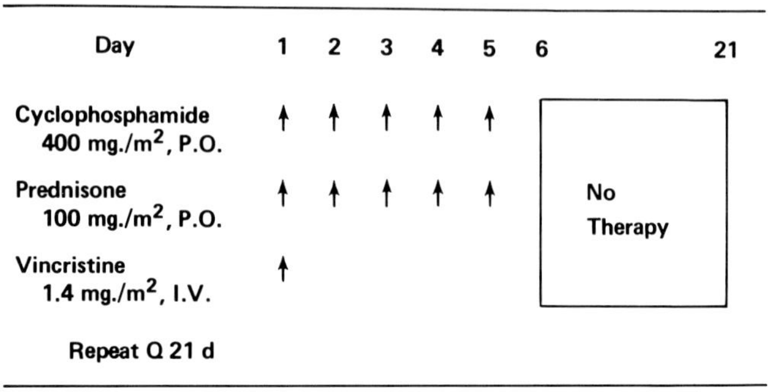

Day	1	2	3	4	5	6		21
Cyclophosphamide 400 mg./m^2, P.O.	↑	↑	↑	↑	↑			
Prednisone 100 mg./m^2, P.O.	↑	↑	↑	↑	↑	No Therapy		
Vincristine 1.4 mg./m^2, I.V.	↑							
Repeat Q 21 d								

Fig. 14: CVP Cycle

basis. A minimum of 4 cycles of treatment are given, followed by 2 additional consolidation cycles, if a complete remission status is achieved. Using this program, 57% of patients have attained a complete remission. An additional 34% of patients achieved a partial response defined as a 75% or greater reduction in measurable disease, bringing the overall response rate to 91%. The survival of the complete remission group at 2 years is 84% and 74% for all patients. The median survival of this study has not been reached (3).

Historically, the earliest successful use of combination chemotherapy was in the treatment of metastatic testicular carcinoma. In 1960, Li reported on the combined use of methotrexate, chlorambucil and actinomycin-D in radiation-resistant forms of testicular cancer (27). He demonstrated a response rate of 50%, with 7 of 23 patients having a complete or near complete disappearance of pulmonary metastases and palpable tumor masses. Several of the patients from this series have remained clinically free of their

disease for as long as 13 years. Subsequently, Mackenzie has demonstrated a comparable response rate
using actinomycin-D alone (28). The drug mithramycin
has been shown to have specific activity against the
embryonal form of testicular carcinoma with a response
rate in excess of 40% and extended durations of remission (25). In view of the responsiveness of this
group of tumors to drug treatment at these late stages
of disease, a chemotherapy adjuvant program in testicular cancer appears warranted.

The most recent chapter in the clinical use of
drug combinations has been in the treatment of breast
cancer. In 1969, Cooper reported on the use of a 5
drug regimen for patients who either presented with
advanced disease or who had failed from previous surgery, radiation therapy and hormonal management (7).
A complete remission rate of over 70% was obtained in
patients who had metastatic spread to liver and lung
which in the past have been regarded as areas refractory to treatment. A similar high rate of response
to combination chemotherapy has now been confirmed by
several institutions (1) and must be regarded as a
significant advance when one considers the prevalence
of this tumor.

In closing, I would like to once again emphasize
that in order to illustrate current concepts in treatment, I have selected specific instances where cancer
chemotherapy has made significant progress. I would
be remiss in not pointing out that many important
solid tumors, such as the pulmonary and gastrointestinal malignancies, remain relatively refractory to
present therapeutic modalities. Nevertheless, it is
hoped that with the application of our expanding knowledge of tumor cell growth to the future selection and
use of chemotherapeutic compounds, the gratifying results presently being obtained in specific diseases
might be extended to many more of the neoplastic conditions of man.

References

1. Ansfield, F.J., Ramirez, G., Korbitz, E.C., Davis, H.L. Five-drug therapy for advanced breast cancer; a phase I study. Cancer Chemotherap. Rept. 55, 183-188 (1971).

2. Aur, R.J.A., Simone, J., Hustu, H.O., Waters, T., Borella, L., Pratt, C. and Pinkel, D.. Central nervous system therapy and combination chemotherapy of childhood lymphocytic leukemia. Blood 37, 272-281 (1971).

3. Bagley, C.M., DeVita, V.T., Berard, C.W., Canellos, G.P. Advanced lymphosarcoma: intensive cyclical combination chemotherapy with cyclophosphamide, vincristine and prednisone (CVP). Ann. Int. Med. 76, 227-234 (1972).

4. Bruce, W.R., Meeker, B.E., Valeriote, F.A. Comparison of the sensitivity of normal hematopoetic and transplanted lymphoma colony forming cells to chemotherapeutic agents administered in vivo. J. Nat. Cancer Inst. 37, 233-245 (1966).

5. Collins, V.P., Loeffler, R.K., Tivey, H. Observations on growth rates of human tumors. Am. J. Roentgenology 76, 988-1000 (1956).

6. Cooper, E.H., Frank, G.L., Wright, D.H. Cell Proliferation in Burkitt's tumor. Europ. J. Cancer 2, 377-384 (1966).

7. Cooper, R.H. Combination chemotherapy in hormone resistant breast cancer. Proc. Am. Assoc. Cancer Res. 10, 15 (1969).

8. DeVita, V.T. Cell kinetics and the chemotherapy of cancer. Cancer Chemotherap. Rept. 2, 23-33 (1971).

9. DeVita, V.T. Chemotherapy of the lymphomas. In Ultmann, J.E. (ed.), Recent Results in Cancer Research: Current Concepts in the Management of Leukemia and Lymphoma. Springer-Verlag, N.Y., p. 159, 1970.

10. DeVita, V.T., Serpick, A.A., Carbone, P.P. Combination chemotherapy in the treatment of advanced Hodgkin's disease. Ann. Int. Med. 73, 881-895 (1970).

11. Elion, G.B., Singer, S., Hitchings, G.H. Antagonists of nucleic acid derivatives. VIII. Synergism in combinations of biochemically related antimetabolites. J. Biol. Chem. 208, 477-488 (1954).

12. Fairley, H.G. Combination chemotherapy in malignant diseases. J. Roy Coll. Phycns. Lond. 5, 167-177 (1971).

13. Farber, S. Chemotherapy in the treatment of leukemia and Wilm's tumor. JAMA 198, 826-836 (1966).

14. Fisher, B., Ravdin, R.G., Ausman, R.K., Slack, N.H., Moore, G.E., Moer, R.J. Surgical adjuvant chemotherapy in cancer of the breast: results of a decade of cooperative investigation. Ann. Surg. 168, 337-356 (1968).

15. Frei, E., III, Freireich, E.J. Progress and perspectives in the chemotherapy of acute leukemias. Adv. Chemother. 2, 269-298 (1965).

16. Freireich, E.J., et al. The effect of 6-mercaptopurine on the duration of steroid-induced remissions in acute leukemia: a model for evaluation of other potentially useful therapy. Blood 21, 699-716 (1963).

203

17. Gee, T.S., Yu, K.P., Clarkson, B.D. Treatment of adult acute leukemia with arabinosyl cytosine and thioguanine. Cancer 23, 1019-1032 (1969).

18. Goldin, A., Venditti, J.M., Humphreys, S.R., Mantel, N. Modification of treatment schedules in the management of advanced mouse leukemia with amethopterin. J. Nat. Cancer Inst. 17, 203 -212 (1956).

19. Haskell, C.M., Canellos, G.P. L-asparagine resistance in human leukemia: asparagine synthetase. Biochem. Pharm. 18, 2578-2580 (1969).

20. Heidelberger, C. et al. Fluorinated pyrimidines, a new class of tumour-inhibitory compounds. Nature 179, 663-666 (1957).

21. Henderson, E.S. Treatment of acute leukemia. In Leukemia and Lymphoma, Holland, J.F., Meischer, P.A., Jaffe, E.R. (eds.), Grune & Stratton, N.Y., p. 47-95, 1969.

22. Henderson, E.H., Samaha, R.J. Evidence that drugs in multiple combinations have materially advanced the treatment of human malignancies. Cancer Res. 29, 2272-2280 (1969).

23. Higgins, G.A., Dwight, R.W., Smith, J.V., Keehn, R.J. Fluorouracil as an adjuvant to surgery in carcinoma of the colon. Arch. Surg. 102, 339-343 (1971).

24. Holland, J.F. E Pluribus Unum: Presidential Address. Cancer Res. 31, 1319-1329 (1971).

25. Kennedy, B.J. Mithramycin therapy in advanced testicular neoplasmas. Cancer 26, 755-765 (1970).

26. Li, M.C. Trophoblastic disease: natural history, diagnosis, and treatment. Ann. Int. Med. 74, 102-112 (1971).

27. Li, M.C., Whitmore, W.F., Goldby, R., Grabstald, H.: Effects of combined drug therapy in metastatic cancer of the testis. JAMA 174, 1291-1299 (1960).

28. Mackenzie, A.R.: Chemotherapy of metastatic testis cancer. Cancer 19, 1369-1376 (1966).

29. Mathe, G., Amiel, J.L., Schwarsenberg, L., et al. Active immunotherapy for acute lymphoblastic leukemia. Lancet 1, 697-699 (1969).

30. McKee, P.A., Castelli, W.P., McNamarra, P.M. Kannel, W.B. Natural history of congestive heart failure: The Framingham study. New Eng. J. Med. 285, 1441-1446 (1971).

31. Mendelsohn, M.L. The growth fraction: a new concept applied to tumors. Science 132, 1496 (1960).

32. Moertel, C.G., Reitemeier, R.J. Chemotherapy of gastrointestinal cancer. Surg. Clin. N. Amer. 47, 929-952 (1967).

33. Nathanson, L., Hall, T.C., Schilling, A.C., Miller, S. Concurrent combination chemotherapy of human solid tumors: experience with a three-drug regimen and review of the literature. Cancer Res. 29, 419-425 (1969).

34. Nicholson, W.M., Beard, M.E., Crowther, D., Stansfield, A.G., Vartan, C.P., Malpas, J.S., Fairley, G.H., Scott, R.B. Combination chemotherapy in generalized Hodgkin's disease. Brit. Med. J. 3, 7-10 (1970).

35. Pinkel, D., Pratt, C., Hoton, C., James, D., Wren, F., Hustu, H.O. Survival of children with neuroblastoma treated with combination chemotherapy. J. Peds. 73, 928-931 (1968).

36. Potter, V.R. Sequential blocking of metabolic pathways *in vivo*. Proc. Soc. Exp. Biol. Med. 76, 44-46 (1951).

37. Sartorelli, A.C. Some approaches to the therapeutic exploitation of metabolic sites of vulnerability of neoplastic cells. Cancer Res. 29, 2292-2299 (1969).

38. Selawry, O.S. (Acute Leukemia Cooperative Group B): New treatment schedule with improved survival in childhood leukemia: intermittent paranteral *vs.* daily oral administration of methotrexate for maintenance of induced remission. JAMA 194, 75-81 (1965).

39. Schein, P.S., Cooney, D.A., Vernon, M.L. The use of nicotinamide to modify the toxicity of streptozotocin diabetes without loss of antitumor activity. Cancer Res. 27, 2324-2332 (1967).

40. Schepartz, S.A. Screening. Cancer Chemotherap. Rept. 2, 3-8 (1971).

41. Siegel, S., Henderson, E., Perry, S., Levine, A. Protected environments in acute leukemia. Proc. Am. Soc. Hematol. 14, 45 (1971).

42. Skipper, H.E. Leukocyte kinetics in leukemia and lymphoma. In Leukemia-Lymphoma. Chicago Year Book Medical Publishers, Inc. 1970, p. 27.

43. Skipper, H.E. Kinetics of mammary tumor cell growth and implications for therapy. Cancer 28 1479-1499 (1971).

44. Skipper, H.E., Schabel, F.M., Jr., Wilcox, W.S. Experimental evaluation of potential anticancer agents. XII On the criteria and kinetics associated with curability of experimental leukemia. Cancer Chemother. Rept. 35, 1-111 (1964).

45. Skipper, H., Schabel, F., Wilcox, W.S. Experimental evaluation of potential anticancer agents. XIV Further studies of certain basic concepts underlying chemotherapy of leukemia. Cancer Chemother. Rept. 45, 5-28 (1965).

46. Skipper, H.E., Schabel, F.M., Jr., Wilcox, W.S. Experimental evaluation of potential anticancer agents. XXI Scheduling of arabinosylcytosine to take advantage of its S-phase specificity against leukemic cells. Cancer Chemother. Rept. 51, 125-165 (1967).

47. Skipper, H.E., Zubrod, C.G. Some thoughts concerning cancer and cancer therapy. Med. Tribune Med. News 9, 11 and 16 (1968).

48. Slack, N.H. Bronchogenic carcinoma. Nitrogen mustard as a surgical adjuvant and factors influencing survival. Cancer 25, 987-1002 (1970).

49. Steel, G.G. Cell loss from experimental tumours. Cell Tissue Kinet. 1, 193-207 (1968).

50. Steuart, C.D., Burke, P.J., Owens, A.H., Jr. Correlation of ara-C metabolism and clinical response in acute leukemia. Proc. Am. Assoc. Cancer Res. 12, 89 (1971).

51. Tannock, I.F. The realtion between cell proliferation and the vascular system in a transplanted mouse mammary tumor. Brit. J. Cancer 22, 258-273 (1968).

52. Ultmann, J.E., Nixon, D.D. The therapy of lymphoma. Seminars in Hemat 6, 376 (1969).

53. Venditti, J.M. Treatment schedule dependency of experimentally active antileukemic (L1210) drugs. Cancer Chemotherap. Rept. 2, 35-59 (1971).

54. Wilbur, J.R., Sutow, W.W., Sullivan, M.P., Castro, J.R., Taylor, H.G. Successful treatment of rhabdomyosarcoma with combination chemotherapy and radiotherapy. Proc. Am. Soc. Clin. Oncology 7, 56 (1971).

55. Wolff, J.A., Krivit, W., Newton, W.A., D'Angio, G.J. Single *versus* multiple does of actinomycin-D therapy of Wilm's tumor. New Eng. J. Med. 279, 290-294 (1968).

56. Wood, H.B. Selection of agents for the tumor screen. Cancer Chemotherap. Rept. 2, 9-22 (1971).

57. Yankee, R.A., Grumet, F.C., Rogentine, G.N. Platelet transfusion therapy. The selection of compatible platelet donors for refractory patients by lymphocyte HL-A typing. New Eng. J. Med. 281, 1208-1212 (1969).

58. Zamcheck, N., Moore, T.L., Dhar, P., Hupchik, H. Immunologic diagnosis and prognosis of human digestive-tract cancer: carcinoembryonic antigens. New Eng. J. Med. 286, 83-86 (1972).

59. Ziegler, J.L., Morrow, R.H., Jr., Foss, L., Kyalwozi, S.K., Carbone, P.P. Treatment of Burkitt's tumor with cyclophosphamide. Cancer 26, 474-484 (1970).

SUBJECT INDEX

210